SOLITARY FITNESS

CHARLES BRONSON
with Stephen Richards

SOLITARY FITNESS

JB

JOHN BLAKE

Published by John Blake Publishing,
2.25, The Plaza,
535 Kings Road,
Chelsea Harbour,
London SW10 0SZ

www.johnblakebooks.com

www.facebook.com/johnblakebooks 🔲
twitter.com/jblakebooks 🔲

First published in paperback in 2007

ISBN: 978 1 84454 309 0

British Library Cataloguing-in-Publication Data:

A catalogue record for this book is available from the British Library.

Design by www.envydesign.co.uk

Printed and bound in Great Britain by Clays Ltd, Elcograf S.p.A.

15 17 19 20 18 16

© Text copyright Charles Bronson and Stephen Richards

Every attempt has been made to contact the relevant copyright-holders, but some were unobtainable. We would be grateful if the appropriate people could contact us.

John Blake Publishing is an imprint of Bonnier Books UK
www.bonnierbooks.co.uk

DISCLAIMER
The exercises and actions described in this book are intended for people with good health – if you have a medical condition or are pregnant, or have any other health concerns, always consult your doctor before starting out. Furthermore, some of the exercises and activities are actions that have been performed by Charles Bronson, but are dangerous and very careful consideration should be given before performing any of them. The publisher strictly dislclaim any liability from the use of any description or information in this book. We urge you to act in conformity with all applicable laws and to exercise caution when exercising, always taking care to eat a few hours before any activity and to keep yourself hydrated by taking sips of water throughout exercise.

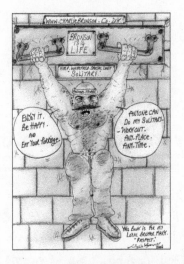

I dedicate this to my brother Mark and my son Mike. You're both in my heart. Max respect, Charlie.

I would also like to thank my good friend Alan Rayment for all his hard work in supporting this book. With me in a cage I am unable to do all I wish to do in my restricted life. Alan did a lot to make it possible. Max respect, brother.

freebronson.co.uk

CHECK OUT MY WEBSITE FOR UP-TO-DATE NEWS ON MY CAMPAIGN – AND
MOST IMPORTANTLY, DON'T FORGET TO SIGN MY PETITION!

IF You WISH To SUPPORT MY
CAMPAIGN FOR FREEDOM ..
THEN Log-ON. AND SIGN THE PETITION.
IT ALL HELPS ..
        BELIEVE IT.
                                2016

Nobody *wants* to die!
So why do people let themselves go?
Why kill yourself off?
Stop and think, get fit and strong!
Even a good shag will burn the calories off and pump
your heart!
There is no excuse – you know it!

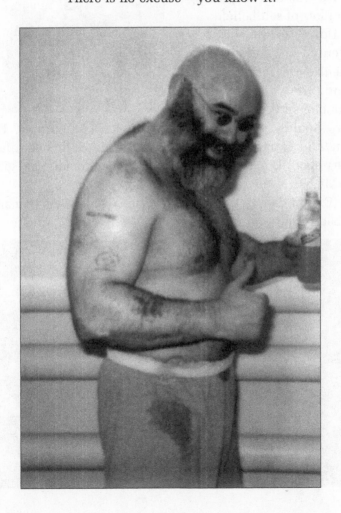

Now believe what I tell you all — stay clear of steroids. You don't need them. Plus they shrivel your cock and fuck up your internal organs. My way will do the trick. Plenty of porridge, and lots of self-belief.

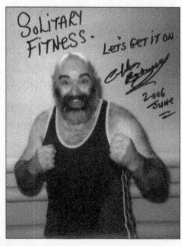

Don't forget to drink plenty of fluids. Drink plenty, sweat and piss it out. And, if you're ever in trouble and you can't get any liquids, drink your piss! You have to survive. Do *anything* to survive. Life is precious. Life's a dream. Life's very short. Don't waste it. And die a good-looking old git!

My best wishes to all!

(Except those fat, smelly, lazy sods who give us humans a bad name)

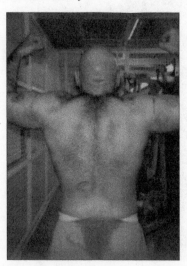

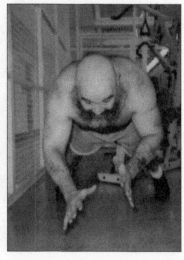

CONTENTS

Also by Bronson

Insanity
Bronson
The Good Prison Guide
Krays & Me
Legends
Silent Scream
Birdman opens his mind
Heroes and Villains

SUPPORTERS OF SOLITARY FITNESS WRITE

ALAN RAYMENT – READING SOLITARY FITNESS TURNED MY LIFE AROUND

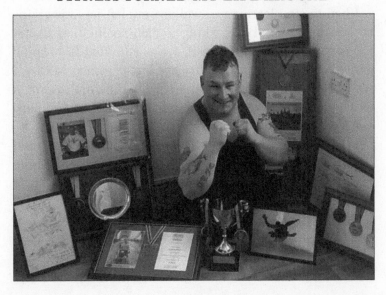

My name is Alan Rayment. I am from Crowle in North Lincolnshire. I am a bilateral amputee and a wheelchair user. I suffered from leg ulcers on both legs for ten years, and then contracted the deadly bug MRSA and had to have my left amputated. What a terrible shock it was to me as I was a long-distance truck driver at the time. Was my career over? I wasn't sure. I spent three months in hospital and in total had ten operations and lost nearly two stone in weight. I left hospital in December that year and that's when the hard work started.

I learned to walk with a prosthetic left limb and everything seemed to be going great. Just after summer I had learned to stand and walk with crutches. It was an amazing feeling to be walking again, my right leg was taking a lot of pressure at the time and the ulcer was getting worse. I was experiencing tremendous pain in my left leg but I battled through. I got a new job as a Transport Manager at the firm I use to drive for and working took my mind off the pain.

I had to stop learning to walk as my left leg was giving me so much pain; I was taking so many painkillers that at times I was not really with it. I was admitted to hospital and told only hours later that my leg ulcer had MRSA. I was devastated: the ulcer was so bad and painful, I was in excruciating pain and I knew what laid ahead for me. I wasn't looking forward to it.

I had my right leg amputated below my knee and everything went extremely well. I was discharged from hospital after only two weeks, but this time I was in a wheelchair. My main aim was to walk again no matter what it took. The leg was healing well and I was back at work, but then another shock came in December when I had a car accident. My car left the road and slid into a drain and sank. I had to break the window to get out. I swam to the side of the drain and waited for assistance. The fire and ambulance crew came to the rescue. It was a cold freezing December evening and I couldn't believe my luck. I shouldn't be here today. My right stump had been injured in the accident and it didn't look too good as my wound had opened up.

The following year I spent working, hoping my leg would heal below my knee, but it didn't look good. I spent a full year with dressings on my leg, and the pain had crept back in. All I wanted to do was get measured up for another prosthetic limb and get walking again, but it wasn't to be. I visited a surgeon and asked him to amputate my leg above my knee; I knew I still had a chance to walk again, although I was told it was going to be extremely hard as I would have no knee joints. I had the operation and my leg healed within 28 days. I was excited that I was going to be measured up for my right leg, and things were looking up.

I had put on a lot of weight and I felt really uncomfortable with myself. I knew I had to be strong and fit if I wanted to give walking my all, and I had to lose some of the excess pounds. I was nearly two stone overweight so there was a lot of work to do.

I asked myself a few questions. Should I go to a gym? Will it cost me a fortune? Would people stare at me? I concluded that I needed a programme I could follow in my own home. I bought a book, *Solitary Fitness*, by Charles Bronson. I had read about Charlie and I knew how fit and strong he was, and I wanted to be strong like him. Charlie has achieved so much and I knew just how serious he was about fitness.

118 Push ups in sixty seconds!
1790 Sit ups in 1 hour!
This is amazing!

I started to read and it was incredible – just what I needed. The book was easy to follow I started the exercises in my own home on the kitchen floor. There was nobody to stare at me and it was free. I followed the book step by step just as Charlie said. I did the exercises every day, sometimes twice a day.

After only a few weeks I was getting strong and I had even managed to lose some of the weight I had gained since being in my wheelchair. The book was like my bible. I swear by it – it helped me through some extremely tough times.

I learned to walk during two years at physio, but I found it very difficult as I was experiencing a lot of pain in my groin and on the ends of my stumps. I had a long chat with my physio assistant and she told me that, although I was doing really well, if I wanted to go long distances I would still have to use my wheelchair. This made me question why I was putting so much effort into walking if I would still have to use my chair. My prosthetic limbs were very heavy and uncomfortable to wear; they seemed to hold me back and at times get in the way.

I made the decision to spend time in my wheelchair and get on with life. I had missed out on so much, and there was so much I wanted to do, and I was going to do the lot. I said that every year I would take on a different challenge to raise money for charity. My first challenge was a sky dive to raise money for Cancer Research. I learned to DJ and raised lots of money for different charities.

In 2004, I was given the ultimate challenge. I was asked to take part in the London Marathon with my best friend. I rose to the challenge and in April 2004 I completed the London Marathon in my day chair, not a race chair, just my simple everyday chair. My hands were blistered like never before, what kept me going was we had raised thousands of pounds for different charities: Sense (deaf and blind people) Cancer Research, Lindsey Lodge Hospice and St Oswald's Church in Crowle.

In June 2004, I was one of 150 people selected to carry the Olympic torch in London on its way to the Olympic Games in Athens. The Olympic Torch was in London for the first time since 1948. 'Pass the flame, unite the world' was the theme of the Athens 2004 Olympic Games. The Olympic Games touches millions of people, irrespective of age, gender, race or religion. They represent the greatest sporting spectacle in the world and for thousands of Olympians the games are the highlight of their sporting career, the culmination of years of training and the fulfilment of their childhood dreams. To be part of the Olympic torch relay was amazing, one day I will treasure for the rest of my life.

I enjoyed taking part in the marathon so much that in September 2004 I completed the Great North Run, and I raised money for Get Kids Going, a charity that helps disabled children.

Then I set myself the biggest challenge of all for the year 2005. I was to hand-cycle 500km over Vietnam and Cambodia. You can read the story of that trip below.

As you can tell from my story, I have turned my life around. Having a disability makes me no different from anyone else. I have a very active life and keeping fit is a massive part of it. I have achieved so much over the last few years; it's taken a lot of hard work, but I have enjoyed every minute of it. I find it very relaxing working out. It seems to de-stress me a great deal, and after everything I am looking after myself.

My work out with my medicine ball

I do a lot of my workout with a medicine ball. There is so much you can do with them, they are great.

I do the following, but am always sure to warm up and stretch first.

Press-ups, Sit-ups, Crunches, Plank, Throws, Back raise, Squats, Side raise

Being a wheelchair user, I find it so hard to keep my weight down, you have to exercise and eat well. You will soon see a difference when you start training and eating well. You will be full of energy, and you will want to train every day. Believe me, it's an amazing feeling getting fit, you never know one day you may be lining up to compete in the London Marathon or Great North Run. I have gone from strength to strength since taking up training and I now train five days a week. I have never felt so strong and healthy.

Solitary Fitness has helped me gain confidence and better health, and the workouts have increased my stamina and mobility. I have achieved so much since picking up *Solitary Fitness*. It is an incredible read. Charlie has helped me so much the last few years; he has given me the confidence to attempt challenges. The advice and encouragement he has given me is brilliant; I can't wait one day to have a workout with Charlie in my kitchen. www.alanrayment.co.uk

VIETNAM & CAMBODIA CYCLE CHALLENGE, NOVEMBER 2005

My good friend Tony Simpson called me and asked if I would take on a massive challenge, one that would push me to the limits. I listened to what he had to say. He asked if I would consider cycling 500km over Vietnam and Cambodia to raise money for a charity called Whizz-kidz, a charity that helps change the lives of many disabled children in the UK. I told Tony to send me the details.

I received the itinerary on what the challenge had to offer and it sounded amazing. I sent back my application form with the deposit to book me on the trip, which was to take place in November 2005. Tony had also booked on the trip. We decided to call the event 'The Asda Challenge' as both Tony and I worked for Asda. We wanted to get a team together so we advertised internally at Asda to get more people interested. We managed to get a team of eight of us from Asda and we were looking to raise at least £3,500 each.

One of the first things I had to do was find a hand-cycle and, after a lot of looking around, I finally purchased one from Da Vinci in Liverpool. I received the cycle in April 2005 and I started cycling the first day I got it, as I knew I had a lot of hard work to do. I entered some races to get used to the chair and in total I completed 13 10k races and half-marathons on the run-up to me going out to Vietnam. I raised money for different charities when I entered the races.

I had a lot of hard work to do in 2005; I had to get fit for the challenge and I had to raise the money to go over to Vietnam. I started training at The Fitness Suite at North Lindsey College in Scunthorpe. The guys down there were great. I did a lot of cardiovascular work and a lot of stamina work; I was training sometimes four to five days a week, which also included swimming and out cycling in my chair. I was finding it hard to fit all my training in, as I also had to work 41 hours a week at Scunthorpe Hospital and at Asda.

In terms of sponsorship, I received a lot of support from local businesses and charities, and I received some tremendous support from work colleagues. Asda Scunthorpe helped me raise a lot of my money – we held lots of different events in store – and Asda UK also helped our team a great deal with all there fundraising.

The year had flown past and 3 November was nearly upon us. I didn't really know what to expect out in Vietnam but I was looking forward to the challenge.

When the time came, we went down to London and had breakfast on the Thursday morning before checking in at Heathrow at 9.30am for a midday departure to Thailand. There were a total of 22 of us taking part in the challenge, and it was great to meet up with everyone who was raising money for different charities. We had a long journey ahead of us, a 12-hour flight to Bangkok, and then we transferred to Saigon, before finally arriving Friday lunchtime. To say the least, I needed some sleep. After a few hours' resting, we had our briefing with the two tour guides Chi and Phat, who were going to lead us through Vietnam, and they told us what to expect over the next four days. The following day we had to be up and ready to start cycling at 8am. We were going to cycle 52k from Saigon towards the Mekong Delta River.

On the first day of cycling from Saigon, we were hit by a monsoon. Talk about crazy weather. The terrain was challenging as we cycled down the gateway to the Mekong Delta River and then crossed it by ferry into the jungle. As we cycled past fields of sugar cane and banana plantations, the scenery was spectacular. When we got through the jungle I looked like I had been in mud bath, I was so covered in dirt. It was so wet, if I had stopped my chair in the jungle, I don't think I would have got going again.

In Vietnam we saw the most remote and poor parts of the country. Visiting villages while we stopped for lunch, the locals were amazed to see me; our tour guide told me they were shouting 'amazing strong man' to me. Our journey through Vietnam was spectacular and I have many, many stories to tell. The weather played a massive part. It was so hot that the top half of my body was covered in heat rash and blisters, and all I could do was try and block the pain out.

On our final stage in Vietnam it started to rain and it cooled me down so much. It was great, but it didn't make what was in front of us any easier. We had to climb five miles up a mountain, the roads were very wet and the front of my cycle started to slip as I climbed up. The mountain seemed to go on and on and, when I was about two miles from the top, I had to stop to put my cycle into the lowest gear I had. Two of my team were encouraging me and, with a lot of hard work, I made it to the top. As I sat on the top and looked back down, I was amazed at what I had just achieved, but the best was to come. As they say, what goes up must come down! The drop on the other side was unbelievable – as I got halfway down I was doing 24mph. Looking back, it maybe wasn't safe but I enjoyed it at the time.

We transferred to Cambodia on a six-hour boat journey. Our tour guide was the national champion for cycling in Cambodia and would take us on our final two-day journey through Cambodia.

We started the 100km cycle from Phnom Penh. Most of the journey was dirt tracks and pot holes, and it was extremely hard work. Some of the cyclists were getting punctures, buckled wheels and one even snapped his pedals. We were surrounded by paddy fields and huge open plains, the scenery broken only by sugar palm trees and wooden huts and at times we saw water buffaloes. The heat meant I was in agony and the heat rash now covered half of my body. I was being pushed to my limits; 60 miles in such heat was no good. So why did I do it? I will tell you. We were doing it for a great cause –Whizz-Kidz.

The final stage of our first day in Cambodia was special, as we had now finished on the bumpy track roads and we had the final few miles on tarmac. It was like being at home. I pushed myself on and started to overtake the other cyclists. They were in shock – the two lads who had helped me get up the massive mountain in Vietnam were following me. I finished first and received the yellow jersey.

The last day of cycling was towards Seam Reap. We had to complete another 100km to the finish at Angkor Wat, and there was excitement as the finish drew near. We passed and visited many temples in Cambodia and they were unbelievable sights, and we also went to the poorest villages on the way. In one of the villages the children were using fans to cool us down, and our guide paid them some money. The poverty was extremely bad. The children seemed to enjoy us stopping in their village, and we offered them pop and snacks, although they wouldn't accept them.

Our last day of cycling was excellent. Spirits were high and nothing was going to stop us now. I blocked the pain out and got on with the cycling. I knew I had nearly completed our amazing journey and I was thinking of visiting the temples at Angkor Wat; I was also looking forward to our celebration meal and a good sleep. We arrived at Angkor Wat around 1700hrs and I led the full team of 22 into the city. It was extremely vibrant. Seeing the temples of Angkor Wat was spectacular.

I completed the 500km in six days on my hand-cycle. It was the toughest challenge I have ever taken part in. My fitness was spectacular and at times I was pushing the other cyclists to their limit. The heat and humidity was a massive obstacle, but one I had to mentally get through and try and block out and I managed it.

I was the first person in the world to hand-cycle 500km over Vietnam and Cambodia. The feeling was spectacular – my team had just crossed the finish line and we had raised over £20,000 to help disabled children.

Solitary Fitness helped me achieve all these goals.

INTRODUCTION TO JAMIE O'KEEFE

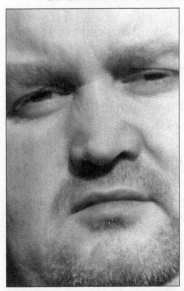

Let me say a little about Jamie O'Keefe so you can see why I felt his contribution to this book was essential. Firstly, Jamie is a normal guy in his mid-forties who doesn't have the sculptured body of Arnold Schwarzenegger types and doesn't claim any expertise in fitness. He is honest about himself and his training needs and is one of the few people I know that took part in my training for reasons other than looking good. With Jamie, what you see is what you get and he is known to be a very proud man who is very choosy and careful about what and who he gets involved with. He puts his pride above anything else and this is where he gains the respect and admiration of others. Don't just take my word for it. Here are just some of the things that others have said about Jamie:

Jamie O'Keefe, one of the most realistic martial artists in the world today, highly recommended.

Geoff Thompson – 2004 BAFTA Winner & Author

One-man guide to bouncers and the art of self-protection.

Cass Pennant – Author & Hooliologist

Jamie's book *Thugs, Mugs & Violence* should be read.

Reg Kray – Kray Twins

Jamie's book *Old School – New School* is a blueprint for the future of security.

Peter Consterdine – Renowned Bodyguard & Author

Jamie looks a right hard man but when he talks he is softly spoken, articulate and possessive of a great deal of knowledge about the human condition. He possesses all the physical skills and capabilities that make him sought after as an instructor but this ability is underpinned by an understanding of the human psyche that sees the 'need to fight' recede into the background, to be replaced by an awareness few of us possess.

Malcolm Martin – Editor, Combat *magazine*

He is also interviewed in the following books:

Ultimate Hard Bastards – The truth about the toughest men in the world

Streetfighters
Bouncers
Hard Bastards 2

He does not mix with gangsters, thugs, bullies, drug dealers, or anyone that promotes these lifestyles and will not be seen at any event promoting such practices. However, you will see him lending his support to people like me, the late Reg Kray, Roy Shaw, Cass Pennant etc who are trying to become positive role models rather than taking the wrong routes in life.

Hopefully you can now see why Jamie's contribution to this book has significance. He is one of the few people I know who actually gives out more than he accepts back. He does things because he wants to and cannot be bought. A proud man, who I am proud to know.

Now read on to see Jamie's honest reflections on the time studying my advice in this book.

JAMIE O'KEEFE

Hi, I'm Jamie O'Keefe.

You may know of my work within the field of doorwork, security and self-protection. I would like to begin by telling you that part of my research involves making sure that the information I absorb and pass on in relation to my field of expertise is both accurate and up to date. I prefer to absorb and test out any new knowledge myself, where possible, in order to draw the goodness from it and iron out any flaws before passing the information on to others. With this in mind, I would like to begin by saying that I decided to take a good look at Charlie Bronson's advice about training in *Solitary Fitness* before I made any personal comments or contribution towards it. I spent over two years doing this in order to check out its contents and effectiveness. The initial 'hook' for me was that I was attracted by the good advice relating to the heart being the most important muscle to train, as well as the section on strengthening the bite and grip with your teeth. Just as important was the fact that it was a drug-free training regime that I could recommend to my own children who range in age from 15 to 25. I am by no means a fitness expert and have never taught physical fitness as part of my self-protection classes, as I prefer individuals to get professional task-related advice on fitness training for their particular requirements. However, I know enough about fitness to understand Charlie's advice on looking in the mirror to see what areas of your body needs working on. I'm not just talking here of your reflection in a looking glass. I'm also speaking of taking a good look at yourself in the 'proverbial mirror' to check out the parts of your body that you cannot see, such as your heart, lungs, joints and everything else that is going on with your internal muscles and other organs.

I first became aware of the importance of the heart as the main muscle that needs looking after when researching for my book *What Makes Tough Guys Tough*. I came across the story of James Fixx – the American running fanatic who could run for hours and was as lean as you could ever wish to be, but died of a heart-related condition in 1984. Fixx had severe coronary artery disease with near-total occlusion by atherosclerosis of one and 80 per cent occlusion of another coronary artery. He was training double hard on muscular endurance and general motor fitness but at the same time it was the effects of years of smoking and consuming bad foods which eventually clogged his arteries and ultimately caused his death. Similarly, I had a hereditary heart condition which took both my parents at an early age, so I've never smoked, don't eat meat and don't touch alcohol or drugs. The only thing I consume along these lines is the daily prescribed combination of medication that I must take in order to keep my heart working. Even with all the care I now take of myself, I came close to a serious heart attack and had to have an interim medical procedure to have three failing arteries fixed. By all accounts, this is a pretty simple procedure – without it, I would have had a heart attack and could have died. I'm fine now but my medical consultant reminded me that I needed to look more into my personal training needs to stay on course.

I was warned not to do anything too strenuous on the cardio level until a period of six to twelve months had passed to enable the stents in my three arteries to bond and settle in. Anyway, to cut a long story short, I took a year's rest from the self-protection scene, built a 'Bronsonmania'-style gym in my back garden and began working with Charlie's Solitary Fitness plan. I took Charlie's advice about going to the doctor to make sure that I was not going to take on anything that may be detrimental to my health challenge, as Charlie advised getting a full medical and a clear bill of health from your doctor, and to only begin the training once declared fit. However, not many of you will pay £150 for a full medical before training. I've recently had and paid for three of these. So my advice here is to check out your doctor's well person's clinic or try to get your employer to pay for your medical – this way you can get a full check-up for free.

Although I was unable to get a full clear bill of health before my training because my health situation made this impossible, I knew what was within my capabilities as I've used this body for 45 years, so know about any areas that I need to be careful with. So, with this all in mind, I set out with my sons to build somewhere that I could train in solitude. Something along the lines of the gym that is mentioned in this book. A very old-school, blood, sweat and guts type of place. This would be just like the old-style backyard gym that Bruce Lee set up. My gym was slightly larger than Charlie's cell of 12 x 8ft because I also used the space for my own self-protection training. However, I sectioned off an area the same size as Charlie's cell to give it 'Bronsonmania' authenticity. I'm probably the first person ever to build a 'Bronsonmania'-themed gym just for this purpose. Not a commercial venture, not a place open to the general public, but a place of solitude that me and my children can work on our Solitary Fitness in. My aim was to fine-tune the inside of my body. I wasn't interested in my outer appearance as I didn't want this to change. People are used to me the way I look so I had no desire to change that; I just wanted my heart to stay good and to keep ticking over for me.

I had spent six months gradually working with various aspects of Charlie's programme, and, to test out the effectiveness of any results, I booked a private cardio stress test at my local hospital. I also had an angiogram, a session with my heart consultant to check the parts that I couldn't check myself. I even had a small camera inserted into my arteries via my groin so I could look at my heart working. And I was awake throughout! The medical stress test included various treadmill tests at different speeds all while I was wired up to a state-of-the-art heart-monitoring machine. For this I also had to stop taking any medication for a week prior so that the results would be accurate and run on a medication-free body. The result was a 100 per cent success. I was fit again. I had three independent stress, health and full medical tests over a two-month period. My consultant, the hospital cardio specialists and BUPU had tested me to the max and I was pleased with the results. I had gone from being a medical disaster to a medical success.

The only physical training that I did prior to these tests were various aspects and drills from Charlie's book that I felt I personally needed.

Obviously I still did my self-protection side as well but this was more geared up to working with skill, technique, speed and effectiveness within an anaerobic time restraint which is the initial slot I need it to be effective. To put it into plain English, it needs to be effective before I begin to puff and blow. It needs to work for me using the oxygenated blood within my system without needing to take more oxygen in. So my personal fitness was a totally separate issue. I don't have a gym membership, don't wear expensive training trainers and have never taken steroids or any supplements. All I used was this book and followed some of the sound advice within it. I don't want to go into my specific routines as its effectiveness and worth will vary for each individual. I also do not want people to use specific exercises just because they are the ones that worked for me as this would not be the right thing to do. To get the maximum results for your own personal needs you must first identify and accept that you have a few weak areas that need improving. Mine was my heart muscle so I devised my routines around that. Yours may be that you want stronger arms or just want to look better. I had a specific health challenge that needed my attention, yours may be health related or simply cosmetic change that you desire. Once you know what it is that you want to achieve, have accepted this and are ready to face your programme of improvement, take on board the relevant advice that Charlie has to offer in this book and take small gradual steps towards getting your body nearer to how you want it to be. If you want to be able to measure your success then don't tell anyone that you are training in solitude. When the time is right, noticeable positive comments will come your way when you least expect them. Whether it's your outward physical appearance or inward health issues that you are addressing, people will be able to see a difference in the way you are carrying yourself. When they ask what's made the sudden change, you can honestly say, 'Charlie's book worked for me. Try it yourself!'

I want to add a few comments here on specific areas of Charlie's training that I feel may be of help to some people.

Yoga: This was good advice which I partly took on board myself. Charlie does speak about the importance of cleansing your insides and ridding yourself of used food waste. Although I'm very into the workings of yoga, this is not part of the training that I personally used to its fullest capacity and also did not permit my children to work on some aspects of this training. Charlie made a valid point that you should seek out a yoga teacher with at least five years' experience before taking too deep an involvement. Although I think that all areas of the yoga advice from stretching to cleansing have a lot to offer, I will fully try this out at a later date. On cleansing the body and dietary advice, I suggest you listen to and absorb Charlie's advice.

Jogging: It's a little-known fact that that in my prime I would jog over the local park for a minimum of an hour a day. However, after having my ankle damaged in an uninvited incident while on the door, the jogging came to an end. After a few years I was able to build up enough ankle strength and support to resume the training. Back over the park and chasing the dog around in the garden was slowly building the ankle back up again. However, one day running in the uncut grass, my foot went down a small animal-made hole that made me collapse, with the full weight of my body pushed forcefully down on my joint. This put me out of action for a long time and recovery took years. Sometimes I still get an electric-like spasm in the ankle joint and it will just give way and over I go.

So, a word of warning here. Although I firmly believe that jogging is one of the best heart and cardio workouts that you can do, and that running on grass is better for you, giving less pounding shock to your joints than hard pavement surfaces, you need to be aware of the unforeseen dangers of holes, hidden objects, etc., hidden by grass.

For long-distance work, I now use a running machine instead of road or grass running but as part of my solitary workout I used a simple 'step' exercise as explained in the book, which consists of a few stacked paving slabs to step up and down hundreds of times to get the heart working. Just as some people would in an organised step aerobics class.

Push-ups: You either love them or hate them. Charlie is the push-up guru so I must add something about this exercise. I personally hate them and don't actually know anyone that likes them, Charlie being the exception. What I want to add here is a little slant on Charlie's press-up advice. If you find it hard to go through the routine of lowering and lifting your own body weight, you are very likely to get disillusioned with your efforts and eventually it will affect you so much that you will give up doing them completely. It is a waste of effort and enthusiasm to end up back at the starting block with a feeling of defeat. My suggestion is to pick a number of push-ups that you will be happy to achieve.

A ball-park figure would be an amount that you would be proud to tell your friends that you do. Let's say 100. It could just as easily be 10 or 30 – it's entirely up to you. Now stand at arm's length against a solid wall, with your hands shoulder-width apart and do your 100 standing push-ups. Very simple! If you do this for a week, then find another solid point six inches lower and do the same again, it will take you about 12 weeks to be doing the same 100 push-ups from the floor. Trust me, it works. I had to use this system when my heart problems worsened and my arteries could not pump blood effectively enough to fulfil my needs when working at floor level.

Self-protection: If you enjoyed Charlie's 'proverbial' cow punch advice and wish to check out other self-protection-related advice, please check out my website www.jamieokeefe.com.

For those without access to the internet , you can write to me at the following address and I will send you some free information on the latest training advice in self-protection: Jamie O'Keefe, New Breed Publishing, PO Box 2676, Romford, Essex RM7 0WA.

On a final note, I would like to suggest that you try out Charlie's advice and take on board all that is of use to you. Certain aspects of the training were not appropriate or of interest for me or my sons, such as training naked, genital strengthening and the yoga cleansing but I want you to make up your own mind about what suits your needs. I can honestly say that I have thoroughly read the book from cover to cover many times before using the parts that I felt applied to me.

The book offers some invaluable advice to any person who wants to work on their Solitary Fitness and I hope you have now taken your first important step towards positive improvement with managing, maintaining and improving your health and fitness.

Jamie O'Keefe, Self Protection expert
New Breed Self Protection

www.newbreedbooks.co.uk

STU CHESHIRE

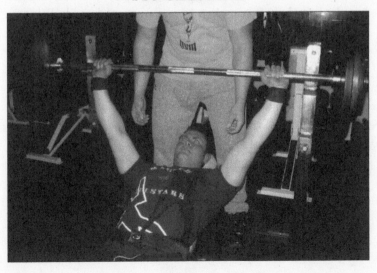

I've known Charlie for some years now and I've always admired his dedication to his fitness. I've trained for 12 years but after reading *Solitary Fitness* my training and level of fitness greatly improved. At the time I read it I was 17st, and very unfit. Don't get me wrong though – I was lifting and moving some very good weights, but at what cost? Too many young lads want to be huge and are training their egos, not their muscles! This is all very well when you are 21, but give it a decade and you can guarantee they will be showing knee, back, wrist or other types of joint problems. *Solitary Fitness* is the perfect guide to pure natural strength and fitness.

On one visit with Charlie, he demonstrated his powerful handstand press-ups to me. Taking up his position upside down like a gymnast then repping out like a true strongman, he knows what he's on about – make no mistake about it! If you're willing to put in the hard work and stick to a good diet and Charlie's training tips, I fail to see how you could be disappointed. Once, at 17st, I could hardly breathe after trying to rep out on dumbbell rows, now I'm 15st, lean, 34in waist, 44in chest, fast, fit, focused and I feel years younger and healthy with it.

A healthy heart, mind and body is easily achievable but you've got to work hard at it. Have a look at Charles, he has the body of a man 25 years his junior!

This book and training regime will save you money too, showing the pointlessness of expensive supplements and the importance of a good healthy diet. The rest is up to you, it's worked for me and I've never looked back. The sky's the limit!

TONY SIMPSON

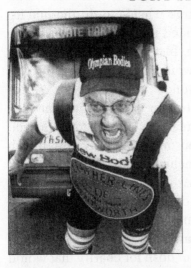

Hi, I'm Tony Simpson.

After reading Charlie's book and making the declaration of commitment, I became a man on a mission and was able to use his Solitary Legs fitness routine. I saw the drawing of Charlie with the man on his shoulders and wanted to make my legs as strong as his using the same principles. I have used piggybacking to do calf raises, as this is the hardest muscle to do anything with, but on the 45 per cent leg press at my local gym in South Yorkshire I slowly increased the 15kg red weight until I could get no more on. I swapped for the 20kg and filled the top rack and both sides till I could get no more on. The next move was to use the same piggyback as Charlie uses. I asked the smallest man in the gym to sit on the top of the leg press, which added another 11st, and I was repping out eight to ten easily. With the commitment promised, I got the largest male plus weights and Neil Goddard, my training partner, hanging off the leg press and managed two to three reps with ease. I did this until my quadriceps at the front of my thighs were bulging out, and was so well sized that, in my late forties, I could enter UK strongman events. For charities I also did lorry and bus pulls. With a harness made by Leather Lines of Wentworth, I thought I was invincible, until I chose to attempt a record plane pull at the Brize Norton RAF base. The plane was a VC10 re-fuel plane weighing in at 105 tonnes. I used all Charlie's warm-ups and lunges, using the large wheels to do the one-leg squats. The thing I really needed that day was my mentor Charlie. If he had been there, instead of only moving the plane about four inches, I would have pulled it off the airstrip and to China and beyond.

To even consider these feats after only a short time took dedication and a book worth reading. When I got to the end of the book, I found a section on the solitary cow punch and thought, Well, I have punched a camel out when it bit me on holiday, and read on. After reading this fantastic bit of info, I used aspects of Charlie's personal and psychological and spiritual methods to my advantage just before a bus or lorry pull of any kind. It was worth it as, if I failed a pull, there was a lot of dosh for charity that would not get raised.

All I can say is that, after reading *Solitary Fitness* and doing it Charlie's way, I found that anything was possible in life. You don't need a gym, but they are an advantage. But, if you are shy or overweight and don't want to be overruled by the big lads on steroids fixes, then you can follow the book and use things to hand from your daily life. You will not go wrong with Charlie Bronson's Solitary Fitness workouts. The book and visits to Charlie convinced me at 48 years old to fight in unlicensed boxing matches which I have won using my Lunacy Pig Punch power.

PAUL SMITH JNR – PROFESSIONAL BOXER

After winning the silver medal in 2002 I was interviewed by BBC TV and the interviewer asked me who was the person I most looked up to. 'Charlie Bronson,' I replied. They never broadcast that interview! Charlie trains without

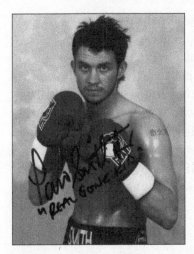

fancy gyms or fancy food and I had to shed over 20 pounds in order to get down to the weight for the Games. I admit, I had to eat all the fancy foods, but Charlie does it on porridge. I admire him because he is so fit and I also admire how he keeps himself occupied by training and breaking world records.

I first became aware of Charlie in the year 2000 at a charity auction when my uncle won the bid for one of Charlie's drawings. He gave the artwork to me and, from then on, the man fascinated me. I wrote a letter to Charlie through our club secretary, Alec McGowan, and we've been writing to each other ever since.

While Charlie has been an inspiration to me, I believe he could also inspire a lot of up-and-coming youngsters when he gets out of prison. I can imagine him running his own gym to help these people with his training methods. Those at the top of their game should also try some of his methods, along with his fitness schedule, and see how it goes. Top footballers, top boxers, tennis players and people from all different sports and walks of life should give his workouts a shot. We might do five sets of ten or something, but Charlie does thousands in one go within an hour. You couldn't think about it, could you? People only see the glory parts of winning, they don't see you up at six in the morning, doing your workouts and running in the snow and the rain; they only see you on TV. Training for fitness has to be all year round. You see people out training in July, running in the sunshine, but you don't see them out in January.

I remember the time when I wasn't working – all the foods you need, you've just got to leave them. If *Solitary Fitness* had been around at that time, then I would have had no hesitation in using the book for inspiration to guide me and to help improve my fitness while on a low income.

I admire people who train and get as fit as they can. I don't think I'd go to the gym if I wasn't a boxer, but I'd still follow a fitness regime of sorts, which would include Solitary Fitness.

Paul Smith Jnr

MARK RAHIM – MARTIAL ARTIST

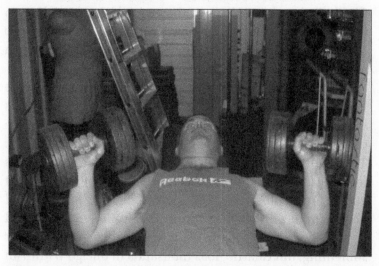

Being a martial artist, the development of the punch is of maximum interest to me, so Charlie's statement that the impact and power of a punch comes from the tricep and not the bicep made me think. As a bodybuilder for several years, all my focus has been on the bicep.

I weighed 18st at my peak, benching 150kg for ten reps without any steroid help at all. Just good diet, regular training and good sleep, which is very important. The trouble with being 18st of good muscle, you find it hard to even do your shoelaces up. To sort this out I took up Tang Soo Do, which is a Korean martial art, first introduced in England in 1945 by grandmaster Hwang Kee. Our martial art has a fantastic history going back over 500 years. I currently study under Master Tony Johnson who is the best Tang Soo Do instructor in this country, training three to four days a week. Of course, there are press-ups involved but I wanted more so I bought a professional tricep push-down machine and 30 sets of dumbbells from 15kg up to 30kg. Another good sound bit of advice Charlie gave me is bag work.

I have dropped to 15 ½st through karate and am twice as fit, with Charlie's advice and training aids; my arms still peak at 18in round. It's not about how much you can press but how fast you can punch. My master's favourite quote is 'a journey of a 1,000 miles starts with a single step'.

So, get off the sofa and, if you haven't trained for a while, get a check-up and join a gym. Better still, take up a martial art. Try a few clubs but go for one that insists on discipline.

As a routine, I do five sets of push-downs with different bar attachments to work all sides of the tricep to get the full horseshoe shape.

A big thank you to Charlie for some good advice from a good mate.

Go on, fight to get fit. You never know, you may end up living another 20 years.

RAYMOND KRAY

When most people think about fitness, one of the first things that comes to mind is how much it will cost. From the payment for a pair of trainers to the cost of joining a gym, and perhaps even the cost of buying supplements, it all adds up. I asked Charlie about supplements once, and this was his reply: 'My 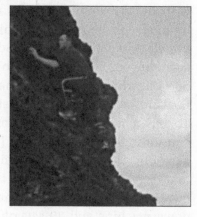 book on fitness will blow all the myths away – fitness and health clinics are a rip-off, so are supplements, so are steroids. If you buy a £300 pair of shoes, do you run any faster?'

I have used Charlie's advice from *Solitary Fitness* for some time now, and with great results, both physically and financially. The book helped me gain overall body strength and stamina, and this was extremely useful when Charlie's son Mike and me pulled off two rooftop protests in London for Charlie. Firstly, we scaled the walls of the Tower of London, then on the second day we climbed St Margaret's Church next to Westminster, and all of this was achieved with backpacks on.

The good thing about Charlie's book is that the workouts are easy to follow and they definitely work. It doesn't matter what level of training you are at, there is something in here for everybody.

I would highly recommend this book to anyone who has an interest in fitness.

SABRINA AND RICHARD MENZIES

SABRINA

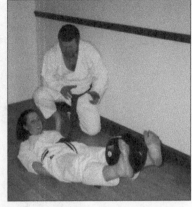

Charles Bronson's Solitary Fitness advice has helped me with my training. I am a student of Sepoy Karate and need plenty of exercise to keep my fitness high. When I'm not at Toddington Dojo, my bedroom is my gymnasium, my body is my equipment and my heart is my drive, pushing myself through push-ups, sit-ups and plenty of stretches. Charlie's advice is simple and very effective.

RICHARD

Charlie has maintained a high standard of fitness in the confines of his prison cell. No free weights, running machines or fancy modern equipment. So, when it comes to advice on fitness, I'd say he's worth listening to. In taking his advice, I have often worked out in my own home using just floor space, a medicine ball and self-motivation. Simple advice.

As a student of Shotokan Karate, this advice has helped me with my training on many occasions. After all, the Dojo of Dunstable Bushido is not a place for idleness.

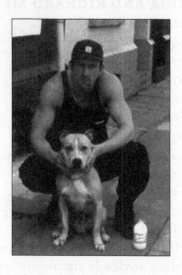

Vinny Clay Bonnar
Shot dead on my mother's birthday, 14 November 2000

Vinny was 6ft 5in of solid muscle. He could have a
serious punch-up. He was loved by his family and
respected by the chaps. Vinny was a Solitary Fitness
fanatic while in jail. He was a proper strong-willed man.
And he's got this page in my book coz he earned it with
blood, sweat and tears. He was taken out with guns.
The cowards feared him so they shot him. In a fight,
Vinny would have punched their noses into the backs
of their skulls, and they know it.
Men like Vinny never really die. They live on with
MAX RESPECT.
IF I HAD TEN MEN LIKE HIM, I'D RULE THE PLANET.
UNSTOPPABLE.

INTRODUCTION

The first thing you're gonna notice on some of the pages is that I'm using a professional sportswoman to help demonstrate some of the exercises. Now a lot of people are gonna wonder why I'm using someone like Storm when we could have got any Tom, Dick or Harriet off the streets. Well, I'll tell you why, coz how do you think you're gonna see what muscles are working if I used someone with little or no musculature?

Storm has trained for many years and is not the average human specimen you would usually come across. The exercises in this book will not give you a physique that will win first place in the Universe contest, but they will give you a body that can be used in all sorts of situations. You'll be able to walk into any gym easily and confidently hold your own with most of the steroid users, while remaining perfectly natural. Your strength gains will be with you for life. You'll develop an inner core of power and strength that will not desert you.

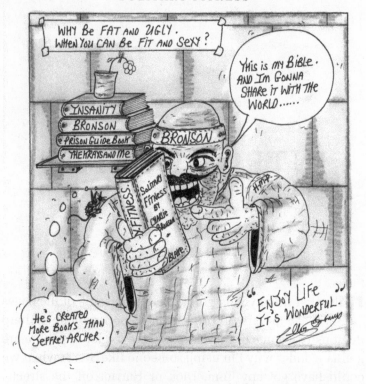

This book is not a bodybuilding course; it is designed to give you maximum strength while helping you maintain maximum agility and speed. There's nothing special about being muscle-bound: I've come across the biggest and best, and I've always come first ... Think about it!

Most of you have read about me or heard of my feats of strength ... all on prison swill! I am the example you must look to; I am living proof that my methods work. I have Her Majesty's Prison Service and the Home Office of the United Kingdom as witnesses to what I say I've done. After all, they monitor me 24/365. No one could take me to court and say this is all a load of lies – I'd call 10,000 prison officers as my witnesses.

SOLITARY
COMMITMENT

I pick up a muscle mag, I start to laugh and I wipe my arse with it – it's a joke and a big con, and they call me a CRIMINAL! All this crap about high-protein drinks, pills, diets, it's just a load of bollocks and a multi-million-pound racket. Steroids ... who needs them? Why, what purpose?

Why buy a £300 pair of running shoes? They won't increase your strength, you're being mugged off big time, so why can't you see it? But who am I to say all of this, what proof have I got in what I say ... Well, read on and you'll see for yourself and save yourself a lot of money. Once you've read my fitness routine you'll never be ripped off again. For the first time in my life I'm going to share with you the secrets of my Solitary Fitness workouts that are now legendary throughout the penal system.

SEARCHING

What do you want? How do you want to achieve it? How far are you determined to get it, coz nothing comes from nothing. To get a body how you want it takes a lot of hard work and when you get it you have to work at maintaining it! But you will enjoy that part. So search, decide and work at it! Don't overstep your goal coz, I'll tell you now, the Arnies of the world really are pumped-up freaks! Sorry, Arnie, but basically that's all you are. It's not only unnatural, it's bloody ridiculous. You guys are never happy: if you've 20-inch biceps, you then want 21-inch – it all becomes very silly!

As I keep telling people, it's your heart that counts, so look after the ticker ... Make staying alive your sole aim. Strip off, look in the mirror – what needs to be worked on? Concentrate on what you see and then make it your business to change it. Within a month on my programme you'll see a real difference, big time! You'll look and feel 100 times better. You don't need a gym or weights, or expensive bikes and rowing machines – it's all a joke! Stop throwing your money away on objects you don't need.

> **Did cavemen use weights? Did Hercules or Samson use a gym? Did they take steroids or swallow pills? Did they bollocks!**

Look back in time at some of the great strong men – to mention one, 'Eugene Sandown' ... well, did he abuse his body?

Being in solitary I am denied access to a gym and not allowed to mix, so I am on my own at all times. I get one hour out of my cell (or cage depending on which prison I'm in) a day to exercise out on the yard, which is a cage 20 x 30ft long! This is my arena; I am the Gladiator! I work out under the sky in the rain, snow, wind and sun in all weathers, six days of every week (religiously) and my routine works: I am a strong and powerful man. On rare occasions when I'm allowed out on the yard with fellow cons, I pick them up. I use them as human weights (of course, with their permission, unless it's a governor). I also get them up on my back and run with them, two at a time. I squat with them, I bench press them – 'bench press' for you novices means lying on your back and pushing a weight from your chest upwards! So I am strong, do not doubt it. My strength is legendary – I once picked up a prison governor and ran with him.

In my hour in the cage under the sky I will do press-ups, squats, stretching, sit-ups, bunny hops, star jumps and I will jog around in between. I do all this to get my heart pumping and I also time every workout, but the most important part of the workout is to enjoy what you do. I laugh a lot. I love it, it's my life! I'm a max-secure inmate. Cameras and guards constantly monitor me. I am 54 years of age, remember, and I am as fast now as I was at 30 years of age. I am 5ft 10½in tall and weigh in at 230 pounds of solid muscle. If I hit you, I'll deform your looks. I can hit a man 20 times in four seconds! I can push 132 press-ups in 60 seconds – can Arnie do the same?

DON'T DO AS I DO, DO AS I SAY!

Right, a lot of the so-called professionals of the fitness game are gonna tell you my regime is based on multi-thousands of press-ups and sit-ups per day, and that this book is gonna be based on that ... bollocks! Those armchair critics couldn't push out one, never mind ten push-ups; they just want you to keep them company ... If people like

3

this are holding you back, they're not your friends. Get rid of them coz they're negative, what I call lemons! Look, even the England manager has his footballers doing basic exercises. I bet you don't get Beckham telling his gaffer he don't want to push out ten burpees coz it would spoil his hairdo!

In order to meet the stages in this book, you'll have to faithfully follow my directions. Some of the seasoned athletes among you are going to push on and start at page 100 or wherever ... Ha, ha! That's no use, as this book is structured in a way that you cannot just go through it page by page. You and they would feel uncomfortable doing so; your body needs acclimatising to my altitude before I can take you to those heights, so be warned!

My workout (not yours at this stage) really starts from the time I get out of bed; I bury my head deep in a bowl full of cold water, then I'll blow out a quick 100 press-ups just to get the heart pumping. Being in solitary I have to keep my mind active so I will pace up and down my cell and every minute I drop and I do 50 press-ups and then jot it down on a piece of paper. You will be amazed how it adds up. Some days I will push 3,000–6,000 press-ups. It sounds inhuman, amazing, but remember, it's killing time for me; it's my buzz! Another day, I will do sit-ups and then squats, and so on. Obviously, you on the outside don't have the time I've got, so you will have to work out a routine of when best to do it, and where to do it, if you wish to follow exactly as I do, but not yet! I'd say do it in the garden. Get a nice mat and you can walk up and down the garden and drop every so often to do your workout as I do in my cell. When I'm bored I will do some shadow boxing for speed and reflexes. I will skip and jog on the spot, I will do some dynamics. I use a towel for this: I just pull at it behind my back and in front; you can feel it pulling at your muscles, stretching – it's a good way of building up. But not yet ...

Sundays, I relax ... do nothing. Then on Monday I am raring to go. When I was up in Hull Jail I had access to a gym for the first time in years. I walked in and put 120kg (2.2lb = 1kg) on the bar – an Olympic bar – and bench pressed it ten times! An Olympic bar weighs 10kg, so the total was 130kg. So what does that tell you? My way keeps you strong, fit as well. The cons had been in the gym for years and years, and even they could not do it. I had just blown away all the fitness magazines and manuals, and I do it all on porridge!

DO IT MY WAY

My way makes a mockery of the fitness world as I do it on the basics. I don't want pills or silly drinks or steroids! Sure, I miss the steaks, but even so I don't need it, so why do you? Why do I need a £300 pair of shoes or a £10 sweatband to look good? My sweat drips in my eyes and down my body, but it's pure sweat, good honest sweat. I want to feel the rewards of my workouts drip down my brow. How many films have featured Bruce Willis wearing a vest, dripping gallons of sweat from his brow ... what if he wore a pretty pink-coloured sweatband around his head?

My heart is in good shape. Is Arnie's? He needed an open-heart operation! They say his condition was hereditary. Let me ask you one question and think before you answer: would you sooner look like Daley Thompson or Arnie? Myself, I'd pick Daley all the time, a natural all-rounder, a fit and fast man I admire. Any of the old-timers will recall a guy by the name of Charles Atlas. Did he do weights! In the 1930s he won a court case when he was accused of pumping iron. The only reason he pumped iron twice a week was to test his strength ... nothing wrong with doing that. That Rambo geezer, he's a superb body on him. You can't knock the man, but can you knock me? I do it all from a hole in the ground on the total basics of life with no sweetness. Thirty years I've survived a war and I'm still on top. I've been to hell and back, and lived in the belly of the beast.

STOP BEING RIPPED OFF!

Fitness and strength come from within. You don't get it out of bottles, the ends of syringes or from the insides of nicely put-together packages. Work out what you will save in a year doing it my way: gym fees, pills, protein drinks, steroids, creams, outfits and equipment? Now get real!

YOUR BODY IS A MACHINE

I see the human body as a machine. Feed it, look after it, clean it inside and out ... Most of all, believe in it and it will respond every time. But like a machine it has an engine and, if you abuse it and push it too hard, you'll blow it up – 'BANG!' To me, that's logical. I can't see the point in steroids and pills coz in the end it's the heart that suffers. Lose the heart and you lose the centre of the machine, it's over!

Once you get to the peak of fitness and strength, it's your duty to maintain it. But don't maintain it with moans and groans; do it with pride and respect! You have to enjoy what you do, otherwise why do it? We can all be fat, lazy bastards, it's our choice! I'm sick of hearing and reading about excuses: if you stuff your face with shit, you become shit – that's logical to me! Eat and drink in moderation, but

SOLITARY COMMITMENT

if you're like me you can eat what you like in moderation, how much you like and turn it into power, muscle and energy. In my book, there's no excuse, unless it's a serious medical problem you've got. And then that's just bad luck; it can't be helped.

I can't really help or advise on a medical problem as I'm not qualified. I can only say, 'Try.' If you're crippled and can't use your legs, then use your arms instead; find a way. If I lost my arms and legs, I'd learn to use my teeth. I do feel for cripples, I really do. Hey, I've seen some of these guys and girls in sports and they are wicked! Have you seen them in the wheelchairs racing around, doing marathons? With one of them chairs you wouldn't need a getaway car! They put a lot of able-bodied people to shame, that I love to see! Respect!

A lady friend of mine is paralysed from the mid-section down but she recently did a sky dive! Magic or what?

PICK UP YOUR EQUIPMENT AND
THROW IT AWAY

My fitness programme is unique as I do it alone and I don't use equipment – I'm not allowed to. I'm in solitary confinement, locked up in a room 12 x 8ft. This is my life! I could make excuses, I could say, 'Err, not today.' I've no gym, I've no equipment, I've nobody to push me, I've got no PT kit, etc., but I don't live by excuses. I do what I do best: stay alive and survive, and if I can do it in my barbaric conditions why can't you do it out there? You just don't have an excuse! You can do it in a park or in your garden (if you're the shy type you can do it in your bedroom). Let me tell you now, you don't need a gym, or weights; you don't need pills or steroids or high-protein drinks. Just how

7

much money in a year do you throw away at your health farms and leisure centres? Add it all up!

Can't you see that they're all laughing at you? You're paying good money for people to say, 'Oh, you're a bit fat, do this,' 'Do it this way' and 'Don't eat that, eat this.' You're like a naughty school kid, your teachers are laughing at you! Well, it's time I blew a big hole in the fitness world, it's time you got the TRUE FACTS from a man who's proven his way works, and shall I tell you what it costs? Next to nothing! I'm not out to rip you off or laugh at you; I'm here to prove once and for all that fitness is all in your head.

BRAINWASHED OR NOT, I'LL GET YOU THROUGH IT!

You're brainwashed by TV showing films of unreal people, muscle mags with images of muscle-laden wooden edifices, magazines full of waifs, or you see a supermodel who's anorexic and suddenly you're the one who's fat and out of shape. Hey, don't get me wrong, I've seen a lot of good fitness mags out there ... but not the ones showing steroid freaks on the front covers! Look at people like Steve Redgrave, that rower geezer ... he'll live forever, while you muscle freaks will die from a broken heart, literally!

There's also too much emphasis on kids to look good in their branded sportswear, but how many actually *do* sports? Parents are partly to blame for how their kids develop eating disorders. I mean, it's only in recent times that anorexia and bulimia became so widespread. Look at Ian Brady ... he'd been on hunger strike for who knows how long, they fed him through a tube and yet the evil bastard still lived on! There are newspapers with adverts telling you that to live longer you need to take this new and expensive supplement. Remember the big rip-off when adverts were promoting an evil-tasting tea that supposedly made you slim? It was supposed to make you skinny as a rake, ha, ha ... Who were the silly people buying this muck, eh?

You see a photo of big Arnie and you're like a programmed zombie, you aim for it. Ninety per cent of you will never become that way as your body structure, gene make-up and bone design will not allow it, but why want to be like him? Why not be fit, fast and very alert? Why not live a better life, breathe better and easier, and feel good? To feel good, you need to look good

FAT PEOPLE ACTUALLY SMELL: THEY FART A LOT

Fat people actually smell: they fart a lot, they're unhealthy and they're sluggish. Look, I'm not gonna mess with you, fat people have got to want to change. If you're one of them, start making that change right now ... not tomorrow! Go to your food cupboard and fridge. Be brave, throw all what you know is useless in the bin or give it to a poor neighbour who ain't got the likes of what you're about to chuck out. You've probably got enough fat on your body to keep you alive for a month!

If you're fat, then it's a fact, I'm not gonna pretend. You're sluggish, you're lazy and you're a joke! In the same way as the muscle-bound Arnies of this world have strained and bad hearts, you're just as unnatural and your heart is strained to the limit, especially like the steroid freak. The fat on your gut is actually pulling at your heart and straining it. Get real – face up to life! It's the 21st century and what a way to start the Bronco workouts! Give my workout a try for one month. I know it will work for you, but I say this to you, don't even start if you don't believe in it. All I ask of you is that you enjoy it, so start now. Eat up your porridge! Hell, I've eaten more than the Three Bears! But, before you start, I want you to decide on something: do you really want to complete this exercise regime? If you want to change your life I would ask you to make a commitment to yourself, a big commitment.

No doubt you've flicked through this book while standing in the bookshop. You've probably thought to yourself that it's full of crap, but you still bought it ... Why? I'll tell you why ... coz if you hadn't bought this book then you'd be in the queue waiting to buy some of that evil herbal tea. Yuck! At least you don't have to eat this book.

SO, WAS IT WORTH BUYING?

You've probably stood there debating whether the price of this book was worth it and toying with the idea of buying it. Well, now you have so you've either got to go through with it or you might as well just send some money to Zoë's Place Baby Hospice in West Derby, Liverpool, England. Rest your lazy arse coz going to the bookshop was the most exercise you're gonna get for a long while! You've probably got a bedroom with an exercise bike that's being used as an extra clothes hanger with clothes on it that are too small for you because you've become fat and lazy. Well, now is the time to get your arse into gear, so come on!

If you're convinced you can see it through then I promise to make a new you, a more confident you, a sharper-minded you and fill you with a new spring in your step. How many times have you promised yourself a new you? You've tried all them horrible liquid meals, you've been kicked out of diet clubs for breaking the scales and you've been kicked out of aerobics class coz you were starting to make dents in the new shiny wooden floor. Or maybe you haven't got the confidence to join a gym, so now's your chance to go it alone. This is gonna be your fitness Bible, the biggest thing in your life, as big as the rebirth of Jesus! But this book is not a floor show for you to ogle: it's 40 years of a world of fitness, 30 years of perfection, even the diet will prove what I say. Believe in it, don't doubt it, you have to have faith in yourself too.

I've spent some time in this chapter giving you the confidence to get it done and now I want you to apply some effort in getting up and finding a pen, coz you're gonna need one in a minute ... So, what are you waiting for? Go find one. For some of you, this next stage is gonna be the toughest thing you've ever done in your life, but if you can do what I'm going to ask then I can guarantee that the rest of what's in this book will be like a stroll in the park. I'm going to tell you something that will amaze you. About 25 years ago, a project was carried out in America. A group of young men were put through their paces and brought to the peak of physical condition, and then they were told to do nothing in the line of fitness for the next 25 years. Time passed and they were all middle-aged when they got a knock on their doors. Each man was given a medical and they were as unfit as unfit could be! Once more, they were put on a gruelling exercise regime. Six months later they were tested for fitness and each and every man had attained the same fitness levels he had enjoyed 25 years earlier! Before going any further, I would ask you to get a full physical and a clean bill of health from your doctor. Once declared fit then you can push on. I don't want you keeling over while following Solitary Fitness coz you'll give it a bad name.

Below, you'll find a declaration. This is your starting point, your first step to fitness beyond your wildest dreams. Have you ever been out of breath? Has the air you gulped for burned deep down into your lungs? Have you ever wished you could push out one more repetition? Well, all I'm asking you to do is sign a poxy declaration, so come on, and let's get started! Anyway, you now have an aim, a target and a goal, so let's go.

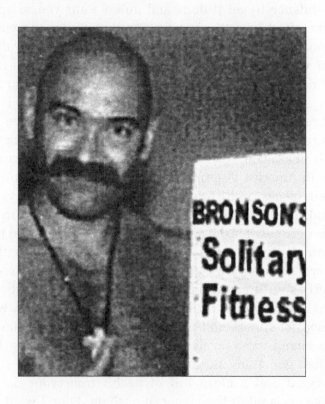

DECLARATION OF COMMITMENT

I, ...
(name)
am making a commitment to myself to complete all of
the stages within this book. I'm doing this because I
want to change my life in a positive way. I've only been
letting myself down all this time, but now that's going
to change.

My goal is to:

. . . .
(Put your goal above, which could be weight loss, to become
stronger, more confident, etc.)

If I give up before completing this regime I am letting
myself down, therefore I am signing this as a
commitment to myself so I can succeed and achieve
my goals. I agree to be a winner because I'm worth it.

Signed . . . .

Date . . . .

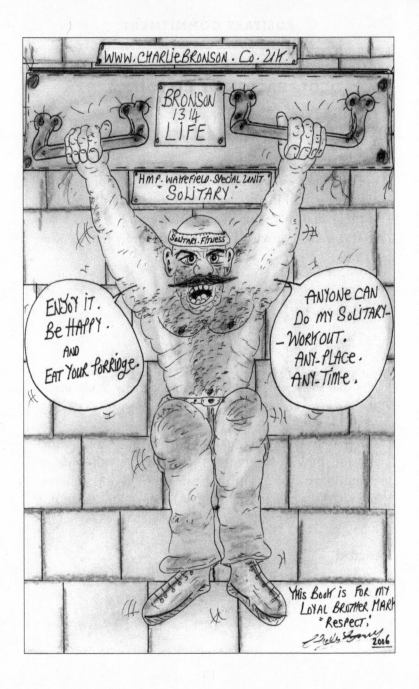

SOLITARY
STRETCH

TO STRETCH OR NOT TO STRETCH

It's great to see you've made a start and there are two lines of thought on this chapter's subject matter. A project relating to the benefits of stretching and warming up before exercise was carried out among many hundreds of members of the British Army. The findings were that stretching and warming up before exercise made no difference to whether you pulled a muscle or not. The Bronco thought on this, though, is a bit different and not for the reasons you think. You see, how is your body going to realise it's getting ready for a shock to its system? If a bull came charging out a field at you then you'd either run or, out of shock, just stand still. It's not always automatic that you'll run or move quickly when this sort of thing happens. Why do rabbits stare at car headlights, transfixed by the light, unable to move, and then ... BANG! Rabbit stew for dinner.

You have to teach your body to learn new things. I mean, your muscles have what is called 'muscle memory'. That means a retired footballer could still get out on the field and have a reflex action to make his body do certain things he once used to do, no matter how hard he tried not to do them. That's why he or she could pull a muscle; it can't be avoided. By stretching and warming up, you're alerting your body that exercise is about to begin and it had better get ready for some action! This warming up starts a chemical reaction within your body and sets things in place in readiness. Your heart is prepared for the sudden extra load, your lungs can store extra oxygen and already your muscles are starting to fill up with oxygenated blood. So you must, in my opinion, limber up.

This saves any strains or pulls, basically limbering up is like a motor: you don't just put your foot down, you ease into it, otherwise you blow the engine up. Your body is the same – you'd damage a muscle or pull and rip a tendon, or even worse. So, use your loaf! It's essential to warm up a bit with a bit of bending and stretching from side to side. I do a lot of high kicks myself to get the legs flexible. It's important that you do it, even more so if you're just starting out. No one is invincible or accident prone; we all bleed so take care!

Now this book ain't about teaching the rudimentary basics of stretching or yoga. All I will say is that there are some basic rules to stretching and some definite stretches you would not undertake at this stage. Certain movements that place pressure on the lumbar (spine) region can be dangerous.

Do you know that if you sneeze while bending over at the waist you can dislocate one of the discs in your spine, or if you sneeze while pinching your nostrils together you can perforate an eardrum? So it's logical that overly stretching can do as much damage without even trying. I'm not going to go fully into stretching exercises at this stage, but all I will say is try stretching out in bed before you get up in the morning. Never jump straight out of bed after waking up: tests carried out on heart-attack victims showed that 10 per cent of heart attacks happened immediately after getting out of the sack, so take it easy. No one's gonna turn up at your deathbed saying what a good, loyal worker you are ... too late! Let your body know what's happening to it. Unless there's a fire, do some stretching before you rise.

On the next page is an example of a very basic stretch. Kids can do this one easy as pie, but ask some grown-ups to do it and see their eyes water then hear how out of breath they get.

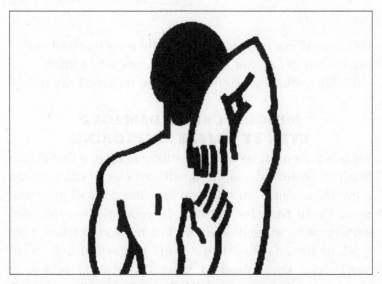

Pass the stretch test! Can you do this? If so, then you're agile.

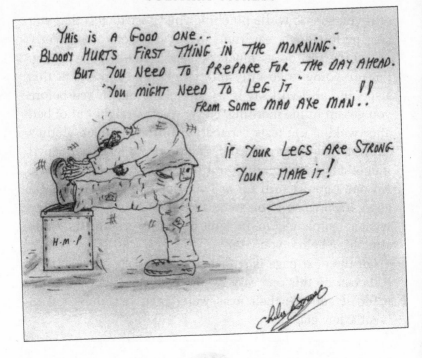

Is this you? For instance, say you did a leg workout and the following day you had stiff legs, you might think stretching your legs would help them recover. I say no!

MUSCLES CAN BE DAMAGED
EVEN BY SIMPLE STRETCHING

Each of your muscles has a sheath covering it, a fine sheath that can become damaged. Small particles of calcium can grow in damaged muscles, giving you years of grief and pain. These particles can only be removed by unwanted surgery so be warned! Am I frightening you or what? I bet a lot of the so-called know-it-alls of the training world don't even know most of what I've already told you: Bronco will keep you on the right track!

WARM UP PROPERLY

An ideal warm-up session should last from ten minutes to half an hour. How do you know you're warmed up? If you're a beginner then you'll certainly know by the sweat on your forehead, starting to sweat is a sure sign. How do you warm up? Running on the spot, running around the garden or anything that gets the heart rate going faster than if you were at rest, even a fast walk (called 'power walking' where you walk fast with the arms held up in the jogging position).

After the warm-up, another stretching session should see you ready to start. Do this before every single workout, unless I say otherwise. If you can, fit the warm-up into your daily routine by walking to the shop at a fast pace and, by the time you get back, you'll be ready for some simple stretching.

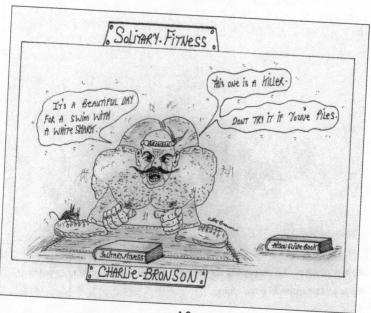

SIMPLE STRETCHING

Simple stretching is touching your toes with your hands without bending the knees, even if you can only go down as far as your knee or lower leg or ankle then that's fine. The muscle memory will take you back to this point at the next session and you can push it a bit further every time. Eventually, you will be able to touch your toes and, if you're really good, you'll be able to place the flat of your hand on the floor.

REMEDIAL STRETCHING

- Touch your toes with your fingers without bending the knees
- Stand up and down on tiptoes

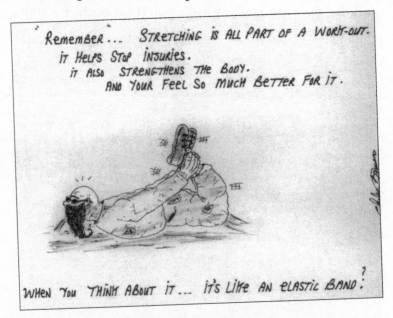

Above: maybe a bit ambitious for the new starter but something to work at. It keeps the spine in good shape.

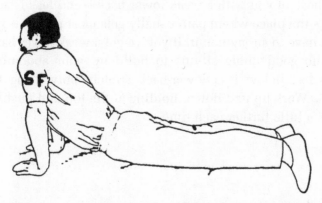

- Holding on to a chair with one hand, bend at the knees and touch the floor with your other hand while keeping your back straight
- Reach out, try to touch the ceiling with your hands and then stretch
- With your hands on your waist and your legs slightly apart, bend from side to side
- Look straight ahead and raise one leg out high in front of you while keeping it straight (hold on to a chair to keep your balance).
- Try to touch your ears with your shoulders.
- Rotate your head in a circle, clockwise and then anti-clockwise.
- At shoulder level, hold your arms out straight at the sides and make small circular movements with your arms, gradually becoming larger and larger, but slowly.

As time goes on, you will develop your own, and more advanced, movements, stretching a little further each time. A little trick is to hold the stretch for ten to fifteen seconds at the most painful part, so long as it's just muscle pain and not a joint or tendon pain.

Those of you with a weak lower back – and let's face it, that's the place where pain usually gets most people – you will have to strengthen it. If you've got a weak lower back, it's no good doing sit-ups to build up your abdominal muscles. Below is a lower-back stretch, only using the arms. Work up and down, holding at the top and pushing back a little further each time.

SOLITARY
BASICS

LET'S GO! SLOWLY, SLOWLY

The governor of my prison wouldn't let me out, so to help demonstrate the exercises we've got the lovely Storm. Storm comes from a solid and stable training background so you're in safe hands.

You've warmed up and stretched, and here you are. Let's now get down to some serious workouts, but slowly, slowly. Don't want you pulling a muscle and giving yourself an excuse to have a rest, do we now? If you've just had a meal then allow at least two hours for it to digest before doing any exercise.

It is important to remember that during the digestion process a lot of blood is working around your stomach and intestinal area. Later on we'll go into the diet side of things. Don't mix the word 'diet' up with 'rabbit food': eat too many carrots and you become a rabbit or look like the Tango man! A word of warning, the beta-carotene from

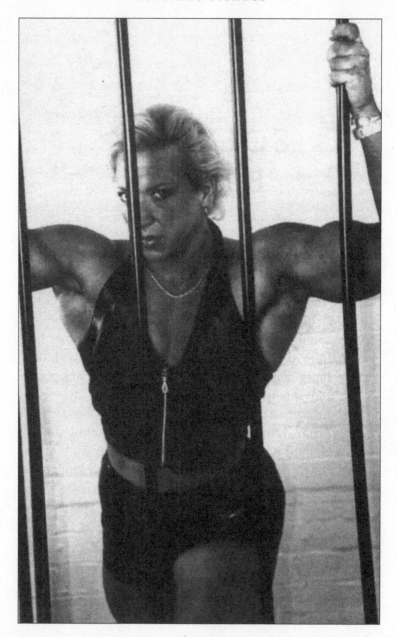

carrots actually makes your skin go orangey coloured but only if you eat lots and lots of them. Pulling the blood into other areas, away from the stomach, is what can also give you a blackout, as well as the feeling of nausea ... Yuck! Don't mix this nauseous feeling up with the one you might get as you advance through the stages in this book when you're at peak physical output. These are the exercises I need you to work on in this chapter – pretty easy, eh?

EIGHT BASIC, BUT IMPORTANT EXERCISES

1. Handstand press-ups (more on this one later)
2. Normal press-ups
3. Sit-ups
4. Squats
5. Squat-thrusts
6. Burpees
7. Star jumps
8. Step-ups

Drink plenty of non-fizzy fluid during exercise – sip, don't gulp!

Start off by seeing if you can do ten of each of the listed exercises, except for the handstand press-ups (at this stage you may not have the muscle strength and you could get injured). We'll work on those a little later on: practice makes perfect! Remember that a handstand press-up is very difficult. You are in effect pushing the weight of your whole body off the ground by the use of your shoulder muscles, while seeing things upside down.

Now if you don't know how to do each of the exercises properly simply because you don't know what the actual exercises are, I don't want you to feel stupid. Look, if you were learning to play the piano from scratch, no one would expect you to know what a metronome is used for (more on this later), so steady does it.

For the ladies who are following this fitness regime,

please don't be put off by what you might consider to be male-orientated exercises. Instead of doing a full press-up, start in the position below and just use your arms. Remember not to lock your elbows out at the top of the movement – it strains the elbows. In time you'll be able to do strict press-ups, so go for it!

A slightly varied style of press-up puts less stress on the lower lumbar area of the back but it still requires concerted effort for each slow and deliberate rep. Push out ten and rest!

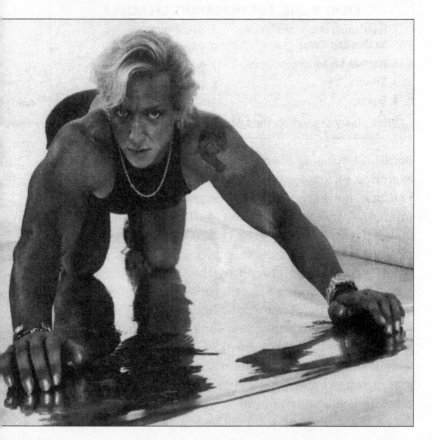

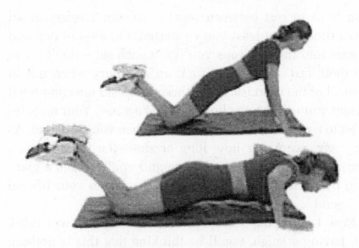

WHAT ARE SETS AND REPS?

We call the repetitions of an exercise a 'set', rather like playing tennis, I suppose ... Not that a game of tennis appeals to me in the size of cell I'm in! Do ten repetitions (reps) of each of the listed exercises as best you can, have a break in between each set, but always try to complete a set.

So, you do one set of ten reps per listed exercise ignoring the handstand press-ups at this stage. This means that by the time you get to the last exercise in the list you will have completed seven mixed sets x ten reps. This is pretty moderate for a beginner but sufficient to test your ability. By the end of set seven you will have done 70 repetitions. A set can contain any amount of reps from one to a million, but, for now, just stick to ten reps per set.

Do each exercise deliberately and strictly, no cheating now. What's the point of cheating? I mean, you're not cheating me, I can't see what you're doing from where I am. But, if you do cheat, then remember it's only yourself you're cheating and not me, Bronco! No matter how long it takes you to do each set, do them the best you can. Even if you have to rest between repetitions, don't worry, it all takes time and at least you've started. Put a bit of pep and vigour into the first reps you do in each set – don't try to do them fast, as you can pick up an injury when not in control of the exercise. Once these exercises are completed I want you to close the book and have a rest. Your muscles need to recover and will only do so when you're resting. As they say, no matter how long or short the journey, each journey starts with a single step and you've taken a giant step by deciding to put the fitness back into your life, so feel good.

Now I know the budding Arnies among you will think I'm having a laugh, you'll be thinking that this is nothing but a rip-off – a few press-ups and few other basic exercises: fine! So, go back to the stinking sweaty gym and pump some more iron, or to your fancy workouts while guzzling gallons of liver- and gut-rotting muscle-building drinks. But, as they say, a quitter never wins and a winner never quits.

PRESS-UPS

Now my favourite: the good old-fashioned press-up – I swear by them. Over the years, I have probably done billions of them, but each session gets better. Basically, with a press-up it's all in the technique.

We all have our own little ways! To the right is a method that allows your chest to go nice and slowly a little further to the floor. Use books or chairs to rest on, or anything you can get your hands on to allow

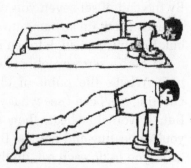

28

your chest to go further and further down. But make sure whatever you lean on is solid and will not slip away as this is dangerous. Vary the press-up so that your elbows bend out to the sides and slightly behind your shoulders: this hits different parts of your chest and ties your chest muscles into your shoulders.

My way is fast, but in control. I love to pump 'em out like an Uzi submachine gun! My press-ups are legendary, behind the wall, but I don't expect you to blow out 100! So, when you hear I do 3,000–6,000 a day, please don't panic coz I have built it up over many years of solitary – it's a wonder I've not worn my arm joints away!

PUMP, BLOW AND EXPAND

My press-ups vary – I do all sorts: wide (arms outstretched), narrow (arms in), I do one-handers, I even

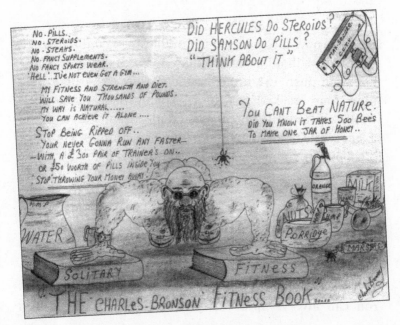

do handstand ones. I do the clapping ones, but all you gotta do at this stage is the normal one. No excuses, so come on! A good way to begin is by doing the ten I'm asking you to do. So what does it do and how will you benefit? It benefits your chest, shoulders, arms and, wait for it, your lungs plus your heart. Your heart pumps, your lungs blow and your chest expands ... Your shoulders and arms get strong – it's bloody lovely, it's the buzz! I'd say it's the same as a junkie gets with his shot in the vein, but this shot remains whereas the junkie's don't! Your shot is pure adrenalin – it's the drug in your body, it's the greatest feeling you'll get! You wait till you're pushing press-ups in their tons! You wait till you feel the flow in your body and the lightness in your head! I'm giving you something money can't buy: total and utter supreme fitness beyond your expectations.

132 IN 60 SECONDS

Did you know the average man in the street couldn't do 15 press-ups without turning blue? But did you also know that I can push 132 in 60 seconds? They say a light man (nine-stone bracket) can do a lot more than a large man (well, you find him, coz it's all crap). All men are capable of such feats of strength and endurance, but first you have to believe in yourself and your ability will come to you as sure as darkness turns to light. I'm not superman, I'm man – flesh and blood – but I have worked on it, I have perfected it to precision. You may not build up to my level, but I'm telling you now, you can achieve your own level; it's in you to do it, it's in us all – strive for your own goals!

When I'm lucky enough to have a fellow con out in the yard with me I let him sit on my back and I do press-ups. You can always spice up your workout, so have fun,

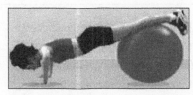

enjoy it! But even alone, like me, you can enjoy it, have a laugh! It's great to do, it's brilliant to push yourself to the limit. Press-ups, I truly swear by them – it's almost a religion to me.

Imagine there are poisonous snakes beneath you as you do it and you'll soon push them out! Also, remember a press-up is chest to the floor, then arms just about rigid, nearly straight – no half press-ups with me: if you're gonna do it, then do it right. No half-hearted attempts or you may as well sit on your fat lazy arse and stuff your face with cream buns! Take it serious coz this exercise is your number one to enjoy. For a good pump-up, use two blocks of wood (I use books). Put your feet on the blocks: this way, you get the full benefit of a press-up as it's pure strength. Hey, could you see the Arnies of the world doing so many press-ups? We don't need anything or anybody; so let's get it done! Now come on, give me ten! Absolute beginners will feel useless but the fact is the average man in the street can't do ten press-ups in the proper way they are supposed to be carried out, arses moving up and down, but no pumping arm movement. Get that chest touching the ground under-neath you: don't lock out at the top coz that gives you an itsy little rest and it's cheating yourself out of the goods you're working to get.

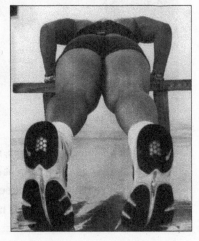

Jamie O'Keefe's two sons have been good enough to demonstrate
four of my exercises for you all to see. I swear by these four.
They are also so simple to do! You can do them anywhere, any
time you choose, and it's a great way to relieve tension or stress.
Sure you can always have a wank to relieve tension, but why

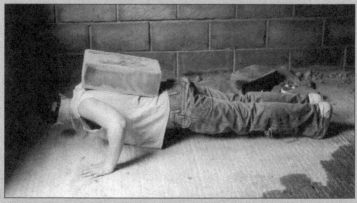

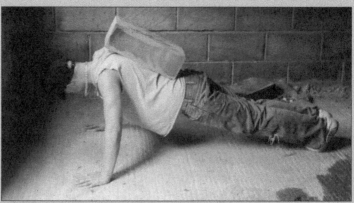

You can do all sorts of press-ups, with weights on your back,
bricks, slabs of concrete, even people. You can also have a lot of
fun doing it. I've done it with three people on my back, and guess
what ... it cost nothing! My way is the happy way!

be a wanker when you can be a super-fit person! All that wanking will drain your energy. Remember, everything is within your mind. The mind is the most powerful weapon you ever have. Use it to your best interest – use it to win. Live and die a winner!

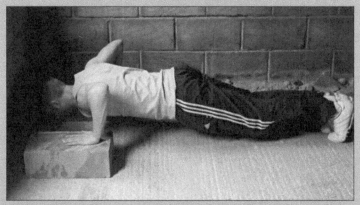

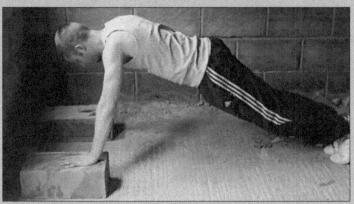

Another great way to do press-ups. This way you get the full benefit. The slower the better. I normally use library books or a cell pipe. I've even done it on eggs ... yes, real eggs! My party trick.

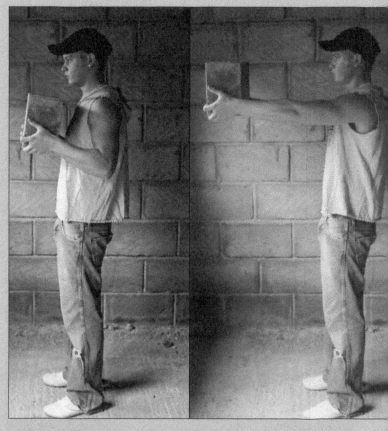

This is a blinding exercise. You can use anything, even a chair.
I used to do this one holding my son Mike when he was two
years old! He's 35 now, so I don't think I'll try it again! Remember,
it's not about speed – all these exercises should be done slowly,
using lots of control. This one is pure dynamic tension. I
guarantee a month of these and you'll put two inches on your
chest. I do 100 with a chair. After 100, you'll have a puddle of
sweat on the floor – it's brilliant.

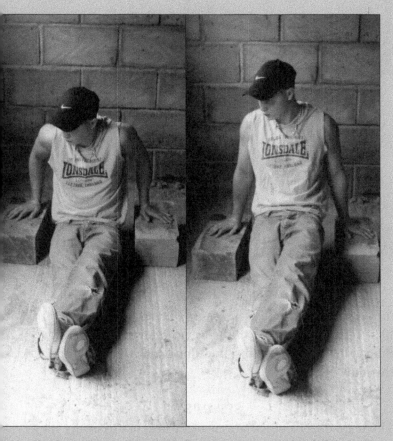

You can do dips on anything. But make sure you're in full control. The slower the better. Do them an inch at a time. Stop. Then another inch. Get the full burn up and enjoy it. Remember you are doing it for yourself, so do it right. Don't mess about, push them out. Lubbley jubbley.

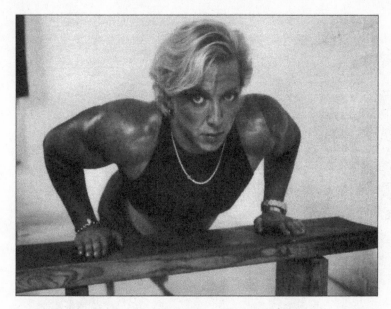

If all else fails and you still find it difficult to push one out, then do the type of press-up shown here, which still hits the upper part of the chest as well as the shoulder. Remember, nice and slow, and don't lock out at the top of the movement.

SIT UPS

There are dozens of variations of sit-ups, but basically they all do the biz. My favourite is 'the crunches': feet on chair, hands on back of head, and go! To start off you won't do 20 (it hurts). It pulls your muscles; you'll love it, the pain – you have to hurt. But later, you'll feel so good! I ask you, how will you be if someone punches you in the stomach? Well, isn't it nice to be able to smile and say, 'Err ... can't you hit any harder than that?' Your belly (abdomen) is your centre: if you harden up there, it will take you through a lot of problems later.

Let me explain to you all now that if you neglect your mid-section you are liable to health problems, such as obesity or cancer of the gut or colon, etc., later in life. Wait till you get to the Solitary Cleanse chapter! I swear by sit-ups: it maintains the posture, it keeps the insides firm and in good order, and it helps bowel movement! Sit-ups are the most essential exercise. Think about it, it's bloody obvious why!

At 40-plus, most men and women start to droop – look at their bellies and arses! It's because they have neglected their mid-section. They have lost what stomach muscles they had and it's just fat and flab, and it not only looks ugly, it's unhealthy, too. But they should never have let it go. What are a few sit-ups in the morning or at night? What excuse is there? It's laziness again, sod it! I think fat people should actually be shot – they are repulsive to look at. If your pet dog got so fat, you might have to have it put down for health reasons. Do your sit-ups, you lazy bastard! Stop making excuses! Do them slow, feel the tension, feel

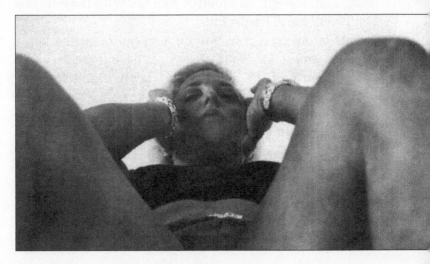

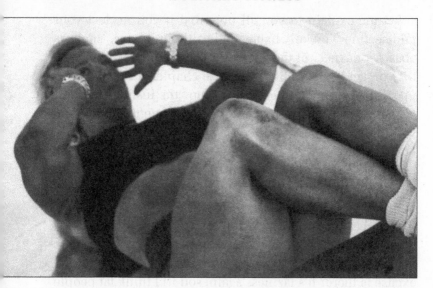

the ripping and pulling of tissues inside. Feel the pain, feel the sweat run down your face. Scream, laugh or cry, just get them done. Enjoy it! Do it to music, do it in the dark, do it in the nude, do it how you want to do it, just do it and stop being a fat, lazy git! Be proud of your body, it's the only one you'll ever have. Respect it!

This is the correct way to do a sit-up. Bend the knees slightly, and once your fingertips have touched your knees, then go back down again slowly. Don't lie fully back down. After finishing the sit-ups, hold your legs against your chest for the count of ten and see how much it takes the pain away.

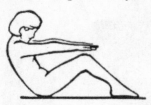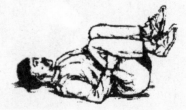

SQUATS

Squats have to be done – it's an essential part of the workout! When I'm lucky enough to mix with my fellow cons, I often squat with one of them on my back as it's good for balance and strengthens up the back as well as the legs. But that's rare as I'm mostly always alone. Start with some pillows from your bed or a chair or a bench. Hold them behind your neck and down you go, gradually building up to bigger items, until you eventually just need to treble your workout reps, but more of that later on. First, just do your ten.

When you do ten with a chair, go for 30 – if not more – without a chair. Hell, why not 50 or even 100? Time is no problem when you're bored or you've got nothing to do! And if you say, 'Err … I'm watching the TV,' I'll say, 'So what? Do them as you watch it!' There is no excuse for anybody in the

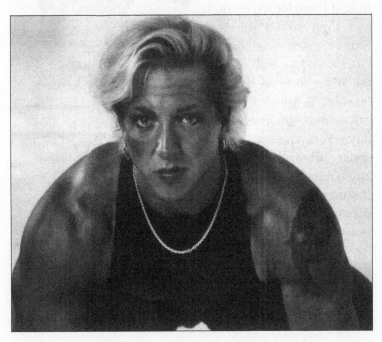

Bronson workout. Any excuse and I will have the answer! So don't play games with me and I'll not play with you. After all, it's your body and your life – if you want to cop out, then do so, but don't waste my time!

Feet apart, go as far down as you can – after time, bring your arse down inches from the floor! Do it in slow motion: back straight, head straight, the slower the better. Keep control (a slow exercise is always the best). The squat will keep your legs strong, so do as many as you feel good at – you can also do them in stages! Go down and stop halfway, hold it there for ten seconds and then go all the way. Stop for ten seconds, up halfway, stop and on and on; it's a form of dynamic tension. You feel it in your calves and thighs the next day. Your power mostly comes from the legs, ask any boxer ... the big hitters, it comes from the legs and the stand; it's all to do with posture and balance. Your legs will get you out of trouble but they won't if you don't look after them. Keep the muscle supple but strong.

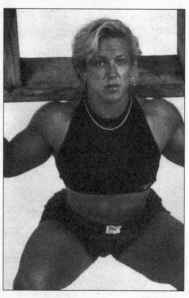

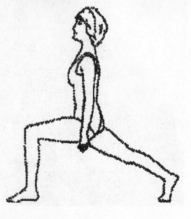

Another form of squat is the lunge. It targets each leg as you slowly lunge forwards, remembering to keep your back straight. Eventually, as you become more familiar with this type of exercise you can hold books, etc.

SQUAT-THRUSTS

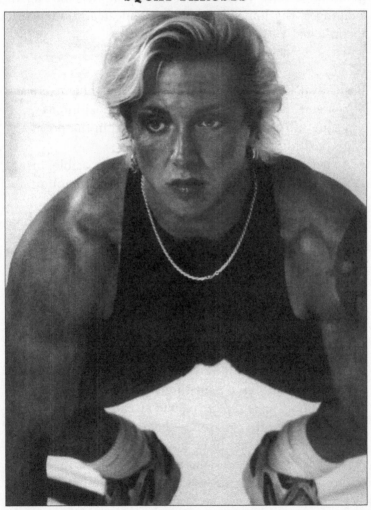

Assume the press-up position, as already described. Keeping your back as flat as possible, bring your feet towards your hands, as above, in a jumping motion so you end up looking like a frog ready to jump. Push your legs backwards and you're back into the press-up position. Ensure your back remains flat and start again, keeping a rhythm going ... nice and steady, no world records just yet!

BURPEES

Basically, a burpee is a combination of two other exercises.

- You start with your body in the same position as a squat-thrust (see the previous entry) in the press-up position.
- As before, keeping your back as flat as possible, bring your feet towards your hands in a jumping motion. Try to keep your knees between your elbows.
- From here, keeping your back straight, jump up to the standing position and on your return to the ground resume the position you took off from.
- Finally, return to the starting position with the reverse motion of the one that took your knees to your elbows.

This is another good heart-pumper, a great exercise for stamina and strength. You need to do these sorts of exercises simply as it's all-round fitness; it pushes you, you'll be puffing and panting and sweating, but it's all for your own benefit, so don't cheat: do it and enjoy it. You'll get faster as time goes on until you have it perfected. The average man in the street can do five without speeding up, so, when you get up to 50, be proud of yourself!

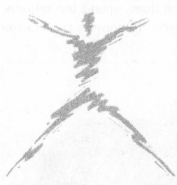

STAR JUMPS

Start in the leapfrog position and burst upwards into the shape of a star. It looks easy, but do ten of these and you'll feel it! A good heart-pumper, it's also good for the calves and strengthens the ankles. The star jump is a good all-round exercise. If you're lucky enough to be able to do it on the grass or a nice sandy beach, then I envy you; it's not a lot of fun doing it on concrete. I do it all the time – it's a major part of my fitness. Sometimes you have to do certain exercises you may not particularly enjoy, but if you're doing it on sand or grass you're very lucky; I'd love that! Would you believe, it's years and years since I walked on grass? The only time I see grass is through a security van window when I'm moved from one max-secure unit to another.

STEP-UPS

Use a chair or a bench – or even a garden wall (anything strong enough), and away you go! This keeps your legs strong. Do so many step-ups on one leg and then change so you're even. There's not a lot to it, it's easy! It's all rhythm and balance – you get faster as you go on – till it becomes natural like

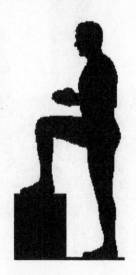

walking. Once the exercises are done, spend ten minutes cooling down – power walk, etc. Tomorrow, turn to the next chapter ... sleep well.

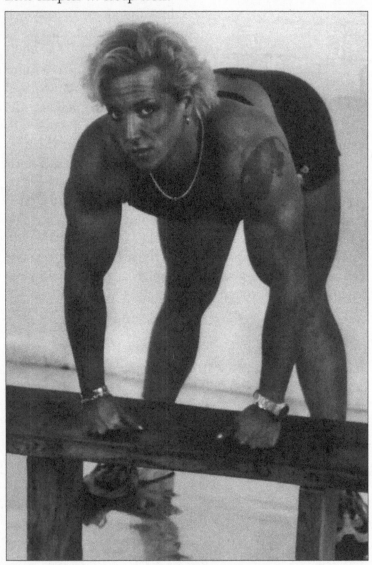

SOLITARY
DYNAMICS –
UPPER BODY

Now I know a lot of you will have started to read this chapter straight away after finishing the last one and what did I tell you? Now shut the book and leave it until tomorrow! Look, it's for your own good to follow my guidance. If you want to mess about, then go feed the ducks in the park coz I don't want you saying Solitary Fitness didn't work for you; I want you to work for Solitary Fitness. No hard feelings, but if I'm to do the business for you then you need to understand, it's for your own good.

Don't forget: sleep is a big part of your fitness. A good natural sleep to rest the body is essential; it's all part of the process. Without sleep you soon deteriorate. Enjoy your sleep, dream of tomorrow, today is gone, it's history. You'll be proud of your achievement.

I always work out best after a crap! It's no good if you're full of food; you need to be light to get good results. You need to work out at your best time – you may be a morning

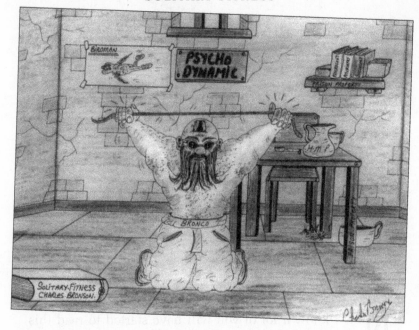

worker, but some find it hard first thing, so choose your time and stick to it.

ANALLY RETENTIVE

Once you're in a routine it's yours; it becomes religious! You begin to love it! And once your diet is sorted, your bowel movement will be regular so it becomes easy to plan your programme. Some people don't go for a crap for weeks at a time. Take it from me, this is unhealthy. Don't waste your time going to see your doctor if this has been with you for a lifetime, unless you suddenly stop going altogether or start passing blood in your stools. For those of you who are anally retentive, I suggest you pay considerable attention to the Solitary Cleanse chapter.

You don't have to be a world titleholder at anything – just be your own champ! Myself personally, I like to attempt the inhuman: I lifted the equivalent of a double-decker bus with my beard in one hour of picking up a 5kg weight attached to my beard. But I almost tore my face off. I had lockjaw for a week after, it tore out half my beard and my neck was like a lump of rock. Pain like never before, but that's me! I don't recommend my feats of strength to nobody: I'm mad, you're sane. It doesn't mix so don't attempt what I do! I've held on to rope with my teeth as men have pulled it (it's why I've lost some teeth). My feats of strength are infamous throughout the penal system and I say best leave such feats to us madmen! This book is about fitness, not madness. Did you know I once squatted with an Iraqi on my back 500 times and I've picked governors up above my head? But that's more madness.

Anyhow, I stress you don't need weights or gyms. If you

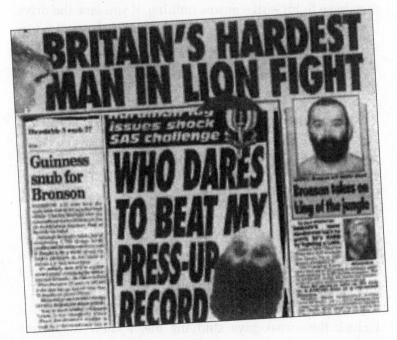

want to get as strong as you can, it's all in the mind. Believe it, have faith in what you do and stop kidding yourself. You're not Arnie; you're you! You'll get faster and fitter than Arnie and you'll live longer too.

Some natural examples of fitness
- 20ft snake – Little mongoose fast, lethal, kills snake.
- Big dragon fly – Little spider traps it, kills it, eats it.
- Big Alsatian – Pit bull terrier rips its throat out.
- Heavyweight boxer – Flyweight knocks him out.

BIG MEANS MORE OF YOU TO HIT
Size; forget it! It's what is in your heart that counts. Stop looking up to muscle freaks. Be yourself: be fit, fast and strong. Remember, the bigger you are, the bigger the area they have to hit – size means nothing. If you lack the drive (and we all have off-days when we feel fed up, tired or sluggish) then pain will drive you! If you're tense, wound up or frustrated then go some place out of the way and scream, let it out!

A FUNNY THING HAPPENED IN THE GYM
Now here's a story and it's got to be told so you can relate to my way. When I was 'out' for a short spell, the Bradley brothers, faces in Luton (underworld slang for the well known of the population), took me to Ultra Gym, a nice place, very popular. I had a workout. I was dressed in my army boots, black jogging bottoms, a loose top, my shades (not for flashiness but for the light – light blurs my eyes) and a black wristband. I wear it not to be flash, but coz I almost lost my hand in an accident.

Anyway, I'm sort of feeling my way about the gym when I clock these two guys studying me. I knew they were watching my movements, talking and so I went up to them. 'Got a problem?' I asked.

'No mate, just curious,' was the reply. 'Well, don't be; just keep away coz I don't like curious people!' I said and with that I walked back to my weights with a strong urge to smash them with a dumbbell. I never liked them flash fuckers – hair like tarts, silly skintight shorts showing their lunchbox, pathetic shoes; very puffy-looking.

Half an hour passed by and I watched them very closely. I saw them talking to the bird on the counter that the Bradley brothers had introduced me to.

These two geezers came over towards me. 'Hey, sorry, Charlie, we never knew it was you.'

'No problem,' I said.

'Er, how big is your bicep, Chaz?' one of them asked.

I dropped my weight and grabbed him by the neck. 'You fucking faggot, what's it gotta do with you? You pair of fairies!'

They scarpered.

Now here's why I recount this story ... I've been there, as big as the rest and as strong. I've bench pressed 500 pounds, but I'm gonna tell you now: it's all crap. Fortunately, I never let it make me vain, nor did I flash it about. 'How big are your biceps?' It would then be, 'How big is your dick?' No, the motto is fitness, health and stamina beats all that muscle. At Hull Prison, I was 18 stone of solid muscle. It's just excess bulk and who needs it? I'd sooner bench press 200 pounds and rep it out good style, or go for a jog or do a circuit. Am I making myself clear? That pair of mugs was actors, clowns. 'How big are your biceps?' What sort of man asks that? What sort of man dresses like them? I'll tell you: faggots, dreamers, flash fuckers! Gyms like that, I don't belong in; they're all fighting to get the best mirror. You should see them stopping to play with their hair or checking their lunchbox is looking good, all watching each other's bodies!

Don't get into this craze. It's sick! All these mugs are spending hundreds on pills, steroids, etc. At 54 years old, what will they be like? I'll tell you: big, fat, ugly gits! As I've told you, train for fun, enjoy it, do it for you. Don't worry about others, how big or strong they are. It's you, your body, your heart and your lungs; you do it for you. And I'll tell you now, you'll have more fun and a healthier life than them prats!

So here we are at day two and you may be feeling sore, but don't let that get you down too much. Your body is letting you know it has had a good seeing-to. OK, for those fancy pants among you who are already seasoned fitness gurus or maybe you just bought this book to see if it would pump you up like Arnie, the laughs are on you. This book is for the person who seriously wants to change their life, so off with you and leave us to it!

But, before you go any further, go to the chapter called Solitary Way. You might be tempted to flick through the rest of this chapter. OK, push on and have a glimpse at the numerous other exercises in this book coz it won't harm you to become familiar with them and learn how they're done in strict style. Solitary Way is the chapter that will become your fitness bible, though.

Each of the exercises is listed numerically (e.g. Solitary One) so they should be easy enough to follow when you are given the instructions from the Solitary Way chapter. Follow what's there, don't be tempted to try out your own routines at this stage. As you become more advanced, then you'll know what's good and what's not good for your body. We all have something in common: we're all different! What works for one person may not necessarily work for all of us. What I have done is to lay down the guidelines covering as many different body types as possible. Your body will respond to my guidance, but after a few months the routines need to be changed to continue to shock your body into moving on. The Solitary Way is the only way – make it work for you and you'll have a lifetime of fun and fitness that will get you through the worst calamities in the world.

Remember to spend at least ten minutes stretching and a further ten minutes warming up before you begin. A good starting stretch is to push off a wall, like Storm is doing below. Make sure you don't push the wallpaper off the walls; keep the pressure on for at least ten seconds or even longer and then PUSH! Now change sides, feel the muscles you're using, try and isolate them; give them a squeeze. You know, like when you're sitting on the toilet and you

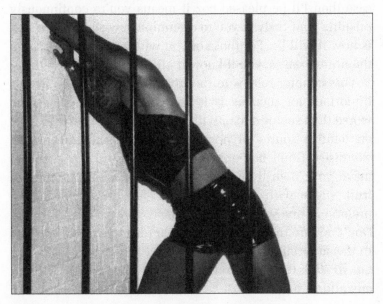

have to give that final squeeze ... Well, the same applies here. Learn how your body responds to stretching and warming up. Don't put yourself into a corner and religiously give yourself a hard task: that will come later!

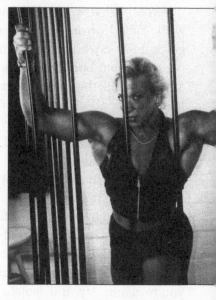

Study the Solitary Stretch and Solitary Extras chapter. Learn what your body can do. Don't expect to be able to make your body do the impossible. At this stage the keyword is 'slowly'. You ain't gonna be able to do all I ask of you, and if that is the case then I'll be pleased coz it means you're continuously pushing your body. If you're a genuine new starter then that is how it will be. For those of you with a chequered past in the fitness stakes, you'll know it all!

This chapter relates to the upper body, which is just as important for men as it is for women. There's nothing worse than seeing a man with droopy breasts! Always have on hand a source of non-fizzy liquid to sip during the exercises. Don't bother with those fancy isotonic drinks, make your own by mixing a couple of tablespoonfuls of fruit sugar with a litre of your favourite fruit drink, preferably one with no added sugar. Sugar is bad for you. Don't mix up the normal junk sugar (dead calories) you buy in the supermarket with fruit sugar. Fizzy drinks make you fat, so stick to non-sparkling, natural juices made without any added sugar.

SOLITARY DYNAMICS – UPPER BODY

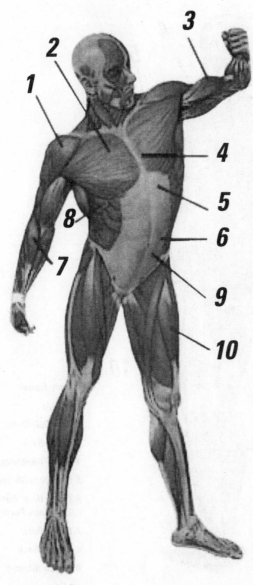

Muscle Names
1. Front Delts (Deltoid)
2. Upper Chest (Pectorals)
3. Biceps
4. Middle Chest (Sternum)
5. Upper Abdominal
6. Obliques
7. Forearms
8. Serratus and Intercostals
9. Lower Abdominal
10. Quads (Quadriceps)

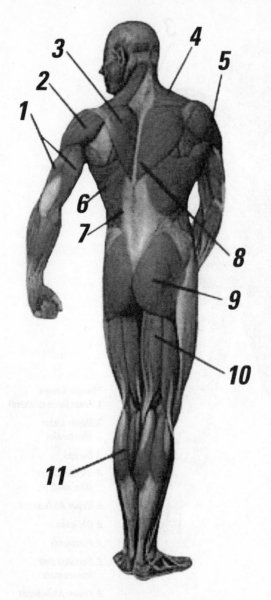

Muscle Names
1. *Triceps*
2. *Rear Delt (Deltoid)*
3. *Upper-Back*
4. *Traps (Trapezium)*
5. *Side Delts (Deltoid)*
6. *Lower Outer-Back (Latissimus Dorsi)*
7. *Lower-Back*
8. *Middle-Back*
9 . *Glutes (Gluteus)*
10. *Hamstrings*
11. *Calves*

54

SOLITARY ONE

Here's an exercise to build muscle! No weights needed. Get a towel, vest or whatever (ideally a material that is stretchy, but not nylon as this could burn your hands or create static within your body). If I've no towel or shirt (often I will be in solitary confinement and have nothing, just a bare cell), I still do it with my fingers entwined, pulling hard and then relaxing, it's the same principle.

Wrap the material around both your hands so the slack is about 46cm (18in) long. Hold it out straight in front of you between chest and shoulder level. With elbows slightly bent, pull hard in an outwards direction and hold in that position for a count of ten. Relax and then repeat at the same height level with your shoulder blades at the back. Again, pull hard, hold and count to ten and then relax. Do 30 reps: ten in front, ten above your head in the same way and ten behind your back: make sure you alternate between front and back.

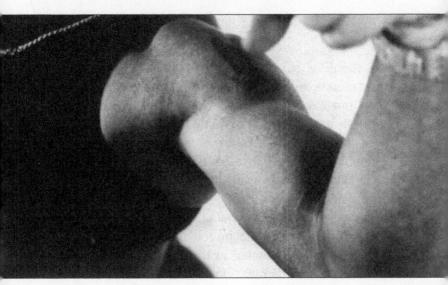

Tips
Don't lock the elbows out, as this will strain your elbows and you could end up with tendonitis (tennis elbow). Use your imagination to vary the exercise, feel the areas it hits, tune in to where it is hitting you.

What it does – This first exercise will rip your chest, shoulders and arms (and I mean rip – pain – but it builds you up!). It will take the blood to the upper torso area, where it is needed.

BICEPS
You're gonna sweat buckets with Psycho Dynamics, as it's pure tension being released, so do it naked! I have to, as I don't have the washing facilities. I find nakedness a lot better to do dynamics, as you're free. It's just body against towel. Also, you'll save the washing bills.

SOLITARY TWO

The shoulder consists of 17 different muscles, all with fancy names. It ties into the chest and bicep muscles. The bicep muscle is the one that seems to attract the most attention and is usually equated with fitness. Next time ballet is on the TV, take a look at the biceps on both the men and the ladies – awesome!

The bicep has two heads ('bi' meaning two). It's no good for punching, as it's a muscle that flexes, so if a guy has a massive bicep it doesn't mean he'll be able to swing a good punch. What makes the punch have a kick is a muscle called the tricep, situated at the back and the side of the upper arm. It is this muscle which helps land a hard blow,

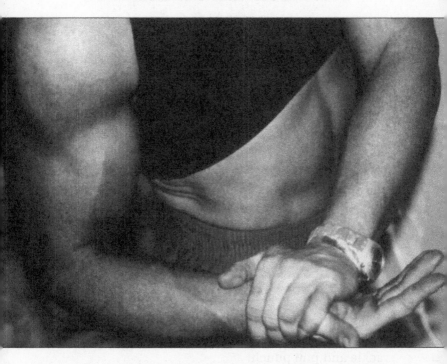

if need be. So don't neglect the tricep: this muscle gives size to your arm, but more on this later. The bicep develops very quickly, so no worries about getting it built up.

As in the photo, hold one upper arm close in to your body so as to support it and using your free hand, grasp the back of the wrist of the other arm. Note the palm upward position of the arm being exercised. Now slowly lift the forearm of the arm with the palm facing up upwards and outwards while maintaining plenty of downward pressure with your free hand and without jerky actions: this is a smooth and deliberate action. Hold for the count of ten and relax. Now repeat with the other arm. Exercise each arm alternatively until you've knocked out a total of 20, ten on each arm.

TIPS

Play around with the position of the hand of the arm you're exercising. As your strength develops, try gripping a rolled-up sock in your hand and, as you lift that arm upwards, squeeze the sock. Hot or what? As you become more and more proficient, you can do what is called pre-exhausting the muscle. Basically this means that you tire the muscle out before the full routine, thereby hitting it even more during exercise. Pre-exhaustive moves for this group of muscles are varied, but a favourite of mine is gripping a sock in each hand. As I squeeze the socks, I turn the wrist outwards and inwards while the elbow is bent at ninety degrees – sure fills the biceps up with blood and gets 'em ready for a session! After each of the bicep workouts, shake the arm to loosen it up.

What it does – It will give the outside of the upper arm the horseshoe shape on the side and help you develop a snap, crackle and pop punch!

SOLITARY THREE

In this exercise you are now going to force the hanging arm across to the opposite shoulder while applying downward pressure from the other arm. Here, the arm hangs differently to the previous bicep exercise. Again, apply constant and deliberate pressure, no jerky movements allowed!

What it does –This helps build the peak of the bicep – it's no good having a massive bicep if it's not going to poke its head out the window! You can have a tiny bicep, but if the head is built to a peak then it sparkles like a diamond. Again, look at ballet dancers – awesome, rocket science!

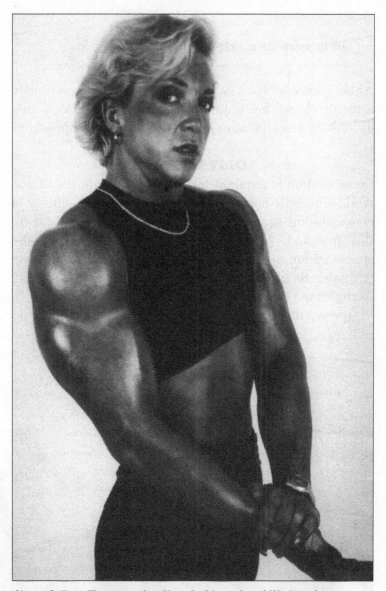

Above, Solitary Three exercise. Note the bicep shape! Work each arm alternatively until you've knocked out a total of 20, ten on each arm.

TIPS
Learn to isolate the muscle you are working on.

Although the bicep is easy to train, it is often notoriously difficult to get built up once staleness hits. Vary this exercise to keep the muscle happy – they get bored easily!

SOLITARY FOUR

Concentration is required for this one: often in the fitness world you will hear of 'concentration curls' – this is a concentration squeeze. Throw away the weights and do this freehand. Note the position of the arm and the concentration applied to the exercise. Get that arm level with the shoulder, lean into it and squeeze the living daylights out of it!

Squeeze the muscle to a slow count of ten and then do

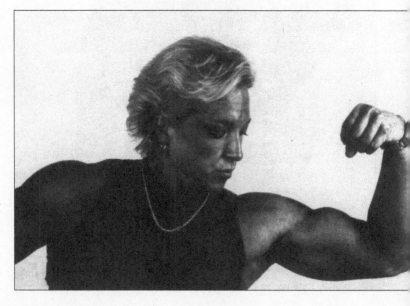

the other arm – ten on each arm will get it going in the right direction. Don't forget to keep sipping on that water.

What it does – Gives plenty of head to the muscle; excuse the little joke I slipped in there! But in reality that is what it does.

> **TIPS**
> Again, as you become proficient, start to experiment with this one. Try it while gripping a sock, let the fingers straighten out and then bring them back into the shape of a fist to squeeze the bicep even more.

In a little book of this size it is almost impossible to include all the related exercises, so I am giving you the benefit of my wisdom. Don't brush it off as being a waste of your time – you've hardly touched on what's lined up for you in the rest of this book! To reach peak fitness, you have to suffer the indignity of doing these basic exercises so you can be No. 1.

HOW THE SHOULDER TIES IN WITH THE BICEP

> **TIPS**
> Small muscles, like the biceps and triceps, can be trained frequently as they need less rest than your larger muscles such as the hamstrings or pectorals. These smaller muscles can be trained every 24 hours, but leave at least 48 hours in between training the large muscles otherwise micro tears can develop in the muscles!

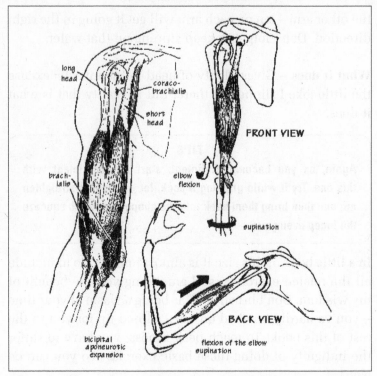

long head

coraco-brachialis

short head

FRONT VIEW

brach-ialis

elbow flexion

supination

BACK VIEW

bicipital aponeurotic expansion

flexion of the elbow supination

You should now be able to identify where certain muscles of the biceps group are located on the upper part of the arms, which is important when isolating them during exercise.

SOLITARY FIVE – DELTOIDS

You should now be starting to notice the names of the muscles being used in their correct form. If you don't know what the deltoid muscle is, go look on pages 53 and 54. If you had to go back to those pages, you're slacking – now come on! As in the drawing on the next page, find yourself a suitable piece of furniture first. If you're lucky, you won't have to use compressed cardboard furniture like me – they won't give me anything else in case it gets broken over something.

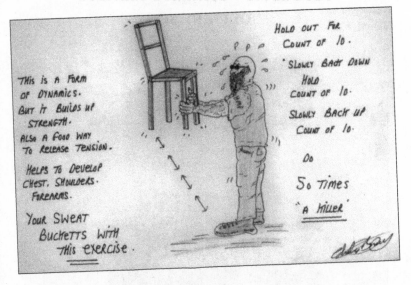

Follow the artwork to do ten of these. Don't let the item touch the ground and if you want, you can grip the item like there's no tomorrow (this increases forearm strength). Squeeze your deltoids to kingdom come, feel the power within you, no matter how small the item!

What it does – Gives a powerful look to the shoulder. Don't worry, you won't end up with shoulders like boulders – unless you overdo it, of course.

TIPS

Start with an item that is manageable and don't use that valuable Grandfather clock or family heirloom! The wider the item, the more difficult it will be to lift, of course, but it's ideal for hitting different areas of the deltoid group. Experiment with the way you hold things and the distance you space your arms apart, isolate the muscles you are using, concentrate.

SOLITARY SIX

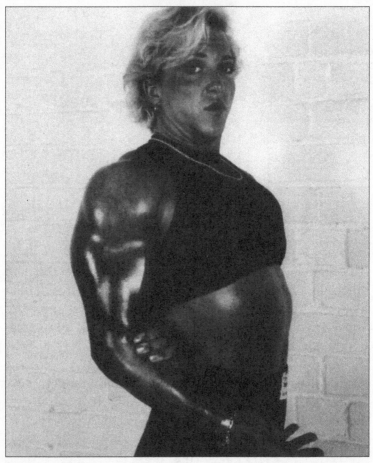

It's as easy as falling off a log! Forcing the arm forward, but stopping it from doing so with the hand of the arm holding it back, apply deliberate and powerful forward motion with the arm being exercised (the right arm in the photo above). Once the arm is held you can give a squeeze of your hand, pumping the muscles up. Don't forget to hold for the count of ten while holding the power on ... rev and go!

Do ten on each arm, alternating from left to right arms. As the old saying goes, 'There's no gain without pain.'

What it does – Creates powerful-looking shoulders, frontal heads get hit, too.

TIPS
Vary the angle to hit the side and rear heads.

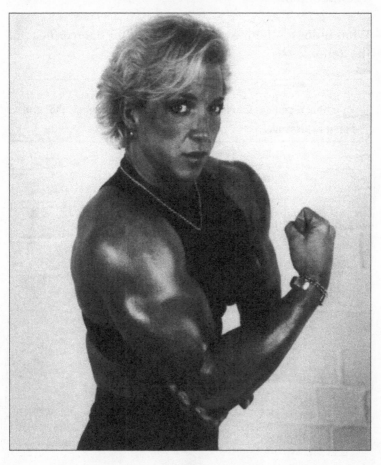

SOLITARY SEVEN

Storm makes it look so easy and eventually you'll be able to exert the same self-control. While holding your elbow, move the arm to be exercised (in this case the right arm) backwards but use your left arm to stop it from going backwards.

Do ten of these on each arm, alternating arms in between reps. Again, deliberately keeping the pressure on in the power part of the move and, yes, you've guessed, hold for a count of ten.

What it does – If done correctly, it will hit the rear head of the deltoid.

TIPS
Vary the distance (closer/further) from the torso of the arm being exercised.

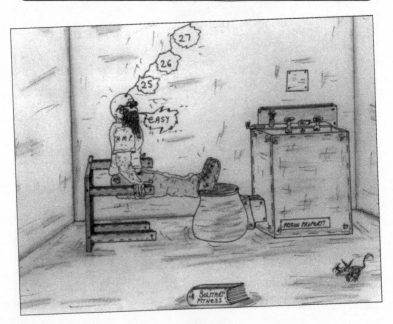

SOLITARY EIGHT

Utilising anything that comes to hand see if you can devise something similar to the set-up I've made on the previous page. You don't need to go to the trouble of creating a prison cell in your home unless you want to invite me for tea when I'm released! Anyone overweight: if you can't find something sturdy, I don't want you snapping the legs off the kitchen table.

Now give me ten slow ones of these. At first, you might not be able to go any lower than a few inches before feeling like you're falling through a hole in the ground. Hey, shit happens – you should have seen me when I first started. I could barely hold on to the legs coz I was so pumped up with drugs (the liquid cosh) for being a bad boy. You don't get the liquid cosh any more, just the cosh from the MUFTI squad with their riots shields and batons.

What it does – Works loads of areas – the pecs, the delts and the triceps. If you don't know where these muscles are then you'd better go and look them up on pages 53 and 54.

```
TIPS
Don't snap the legs or you're in trouble!
```

SOLITARY NINE – ROTATOR CUFF

A very important piece of tackle is the rotator cuff, which is located beneath the deltoid muscle. The humerus (bone) would not remain in place during shoulder movements without assistance from these rotator cuff muscles and tendons, so give them the treatment.

Do ten on each arm as shown, alternating from left to right and holding for the count of ten at the point of most resistance. After a month, up it to 15 reps and so on. Please have faith in this as it will work! It can't but work if you work at it. After a workout you'll feel so good, proud and a better person. Remember lots of people would love to be able to do it but they can't, as they're sick, so you're lucky to do it. By now you should be starting to identify the muscle groups when doing specific exercises. You have to feel the muscle working, feel it moving as you squeeze it. It's a point- less exercise if, when you are trying to train the deltoid region, you end up tensing your whole body.

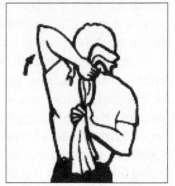

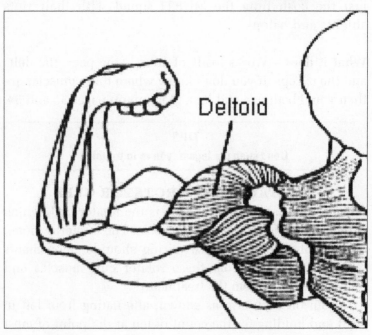

Deltoid

SOLITARY TEN –TRICEPS

While raising the left forearm from the elbow, as below, apply a concerted downward pressure from the right hand. This will hit the tricep of the left arm. Do ten reps on each arm, alternating between left and right arms.

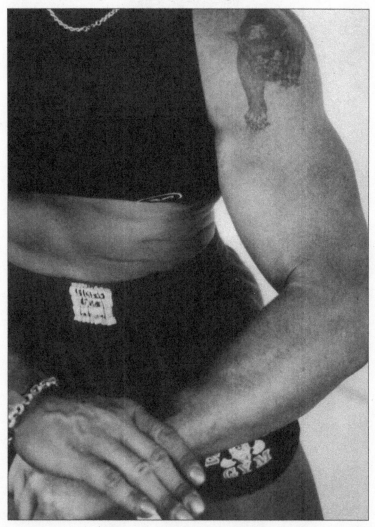

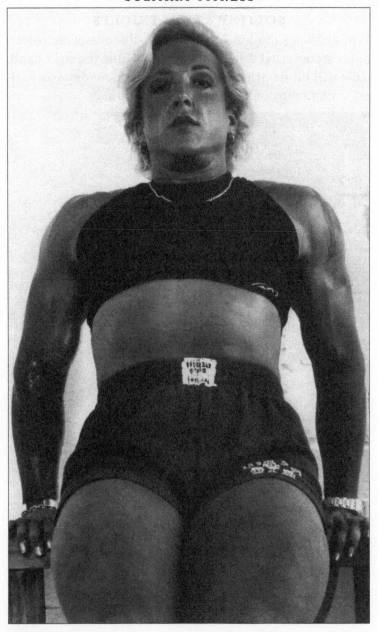

SOLITARY ELEVEN – TRICEPS

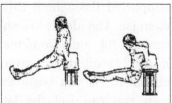

Do not mix this up with the Solitary Eight exercise. Note the difference in the hand position and the position of the legs, which are on the ground.

If carried out correctly, a good triceps exercise will build shapely and reliable muscles. It might seem like an ordinary exercise with little value, but when you consider that you're moving half your body weight with just the power of the triceps you can see just how good this exercise is. There are many variations on how to do this, so be comfortable in how far you lower yourself and don't lock out at the top of the movement.

Do ten reps, slowly. When the arms are almost locked out, hold for a slow count of ten and then lower down slowly.

What it does – Hits the triceps with a vengeance!

TIPS

Lean back a little to put the stress on the triceps otherwise the shoulders and chest can take the strain. You need to hit the triceps, not the shoulders (delts).

SOLITARY TWELVE – LATS

These large triangular muscles are often overlooked, yet they give the torso the illusion of width. They extend from the sacral, lumbar and lower thoracic vertebrae to the armpits. Learning how to isolate this particular muscle means this is quite a difficult exercise to carry out, but with time you will be able to do so.

71

Keep the head well supported throughout this exercise. The idea is to lean over to the side from the midriff section of your abdomen. As you begin to lean you can feel the lat muscle starting to be pulled, so keep the stretch on and, with deliberate pressure, try to stretch the lat and hold for the slow count of ten.

Sitting with your back straight, do ten on each side, alternating between sides.

What it does – Stretches the lats to give that classic wing shape.

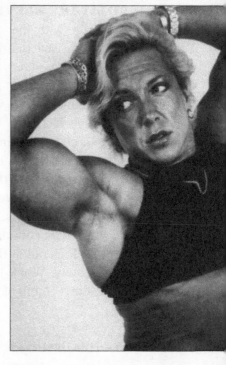

TIPS

Don't fight with your neck muscles during this particular exercise. The hand supporting the head is used to keep it level with your torso as it bends to the side.

MUSCLE GROUPS

Chest – Contracting the muscles of the shoulder joint is the main function of the chest. The predominant muscle of the chest region is the pectoralis major. The pectoral group can be separated into three sections: upper, middle and lower. A secondary muscle in the chest is the serratus anterior (this is the piece that runs along the rib cage). The serratus anterior protracts the scapula (shoulder blade); the muscle can be developed with particular effort but, unless it's exposed by shedding excess body fat, it will always be like a hidden gem!

The chest is the centre or source of several movement patterns of the shoulder joint. There are seven primary movements possible at the shoulder joint:

- Abduction
- Adduction
- Extensions
- Flexion
- Medial rotator
- Lateral rotation
- Circumflexion

Bicep – This group consists of four muscles: brachii, brachialis, brachioradialis and pronator teres. These muscles are responsible for flexion of the elbow. Turn your wrist around and feel the bicep group of muscles work. Experiment with different wrist positions to help you define the best position to have them in when exercising the bicep.

Now some relevant terminologies explained – 'pronation' describes the movement of internally rotating the ulna and radius from the elbow joint, moving towards palm-down position. 'Supination' is the name given to the movement of externally rotating the bones (the ulna and radius) of the lower arm from the elbow joint, moving the hand towards palm-up position.

Believe it or not, each of the four muscles has a function! The biceps brachii – flexion of the elbow joint, supination of the arm.

The brachialis – flexion of the elbow joint; primary mover in pronated position.

73

The brachioradialis – flexion of the elbow joint.

The pronator teres – flexion of the elbow joint, pronation of the arm.

Deltoid – This is a three-headed monster of a muscle. The deltoid works in co-ordination with the rotator cuff to move the upper arm in the motions of pushing, pulling and rotating. These movements are able to occur due to the freely moving shoulder joint. Without the deltoid working properly, you would have difficulty in moving the upper arm. It is responsible for abduction, flexion and extension of the upper arm.

I call this a monster muscle because it has three different heads. The heads of the deltoid refer to its multipennate construction. The frontal head slopes over the front side of the shoulder complex, while the lateral head runs down the side of the shoulder complex and the rear head slopes down horizontally on the rear part of the shoulder. Each of the heads does a different job:

- Adduction (frontal head)
- Abduction (lateral head)
- Extensions (frontal head)
- Flexion (frontal head)
- Medial rotation (frontal head)
- Lateral rotation (rear head)

Rotator cuff – This is located beneath the deltoid muscle in the shoulder region. The four muscles making up the rotator cuff are the supraspinatus, infraspinatus, teres minor and subscapularis. Among the functions of the rotator cuff are to lend support and provide stability in the shoulder joint. This muscle actually holds the bone in the upper arm (humerus) in place within the glenohumeral joint of the shoulder. The glenohumeral joint sits in a very shallow socket; the humerus would not remain in place during shoulder movements without assistance from these rotator cuff muscles and tendons.

The other function of this muscle is to provide the rotational movements of the shoulder joint. These muscles perform three movements:
- Lateral rotation (infraspinatus, teres minor)
- Medial rotation (subscapularis)
- Abduction (supraspinatus)

By paying attention to the rotator cuff now, you will be doing yourself a great service later in life.

Triceps – As the biceps flexes the arm at the elbow, the job of the triceps is to extend the arm at the elbow joint, which gives power to your punch. Located on the back of the upper arm, the triceps is composed of four muscles: triceps brachii (lateral head), triceps brachii (medial head), triceps brachii (long head) and the anconeus.

The three heads refer to regions of the same muscle, the triceps brachii. The lateral head is located on the lateral side of the upper arm, while the long head inserts into the scapula and runs down the arm to end in the middle of the upper arm at the common tendon. The medial head picks up where the long head ends and inserts at the elbow joint. Together, these four muscles function to create the following movement of extensions at the elbow joint:
- Triceps brachii – lateral head-extension
- Triceps brachii – medial head-extensions
- Triceps brachii – long head-extensions
- Anconeus – extensions

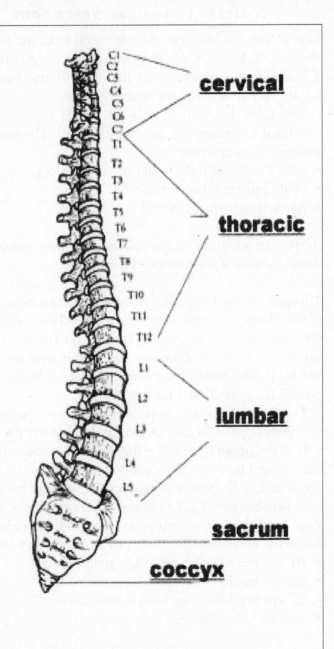

cervical

thoracic

lumbar

sacrum

coccyx

C1
C2
C3
C4
C5
C6
C7
T1
T2
T3
T4
T5
T6
T7
T8
T9
T10
T11
T12
L1
L2
L3
L4
L5

SOLITARY DYNAMICS – BACK

This is all you've got between you and a wheelchair! Frightening, isn't it?

The spinal column is very special and without the muscles being strong enough to support it, then it might as well be made of rubber! Although the discs are lubricated, in old age the shock absorbers can wear down. There is a way to stop this process, but no known way of reversing it, so be warned! When it comes to twisting exercises, there are two rules of thought on the back. Some experts say it is advisable to exercise the muscles, while others believe such twisting exercises can damage the spine. Personally, I'm no expert on the spine, so I have to leave it to your own judgement. All I will say is that you should seek medical opinion as to whether your back is strong enough to go through such exercises.

I have not included such 'twisting' exercises in this book so you needn't worry about doing any of the exercises. The spine is used to moving in a linear motion, being pulled and compressed, but twisting is an out-of-the-ordinary movement. OK, you look over your shoulder when looking behind you, but don't supinate your spine by spinning around from the waist upwards or it could go pop. When bending down to pick items up from the floor, always bend at the knees to take the stress off the back.

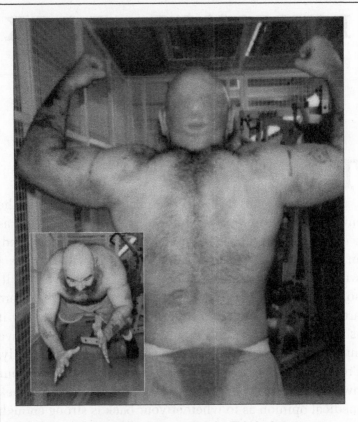

You don't get a back like mine overnight. This is down to my press ups and my dynamics. That's a 54 year old back!

SOLITARY THIRTEEN

Grasp hold of something overhead, as in the opening photo of this chapter. Make sure it's not something that's going to come away from where's it's fastened and be sure it will support your weight. Slowly allow your legs to loosen at the hip and knee joints. Grip your hands tightly without taking all of your body weight; feel the upper back being stretched. At the height of the stretch, hold for a slow count of ten and then support yourself with the power of your legs. Do ten of these.

What it does – Hits the latissimus dorsi, trapeziums and rear deltoids.

TIPS

Experiment by increasing the width of your hands away from each other. The wider they are apart, the more the stretch hits the lower outer back. This is not a pull-up exercise and should not be mixed up with that type of exercise.

Let me tell you about the 'headstand', an exercise I do to help strengthen the neck and the spine. It's not demonstrated in this book because it's dangerous and I don't want anyone with a weak neck ending up in a wheelchair, so sit back while I tell you this story. Some years ago, I actually did this exercise on the edge of an 18-storey block of flats, but that's me. In times of boredom, I do love to test my nerve. Some will say I'm best safely locked away and they may be right, but my fitness and strength are legendary. I'm just sharing with you some of my workouts and it's only thanks to my editor, Steve Richards, that you're reading this, as it was he who suggested I share it with my readers!

The headstand is an advanced exercise and for that reason I wouldn't expect anyone with less than a full 12 months of doing Solitary Fitness to attempt it. Even then I would advise extreme caution. Maybe if this book does well then I'll come up with book two – *Solitary Fitness Advanced*. For now, I have to get you into shape; that's my goal. I've already achieved fitness and superhuman strength, but now I want to share some of my secrets with you. When I start to receive letters telling me how I've helped you then that will be sufficient reward for me.

SOLITARY FOURTEEN

Here, we see Storm showing off her rear deltoids. Put your hands on the small of your back and slowly pull your shoulders back and you should find that this movement

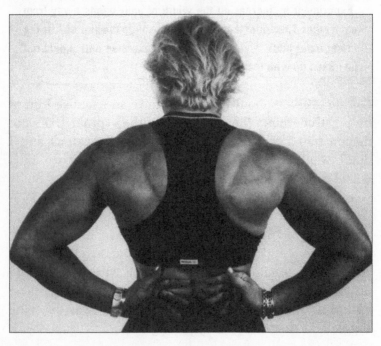

isolates your rear delts. Feel the delts starting to squeeze together. Imagine you have a giant coconut stuck in the middle of your back and you have to bring your delts together to crack it open.

Of course your intention is to get the squeeze on the coconut that just doesn't want to crack open, no matter how hard you squeeze. But this doesn't mean you have to give yourself a hernia by squeezing your intestines out of your rear end! Once the squeeze is on, hold it for the slow count of ten and relax. Give me ten reps of this.

What it does? It shapes the back nicely but, if you don't breathe properly, it can make you blue in the face!

SOLITARY FIFTEEN

By this stage you should be starting to learn how to isolate your muscles. This exercise is a little tricky, though, when it comes to learning which muscle it hits. If it's incorrectly done, you can end up exercising a lot of different muscles. Look at Storm's lower outer-back to see the latissimus dorsi. If you're still not sure where it is, go back to page 54 to find out.

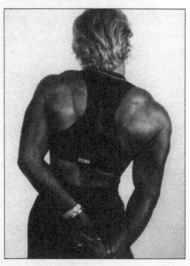

This is the muscle you're going to contract and by pulling at the right hand you will apply steady pressure. The aim is to keep the lat tensed. Give me ten of these on each side. Hold and squeeze for a ten count.

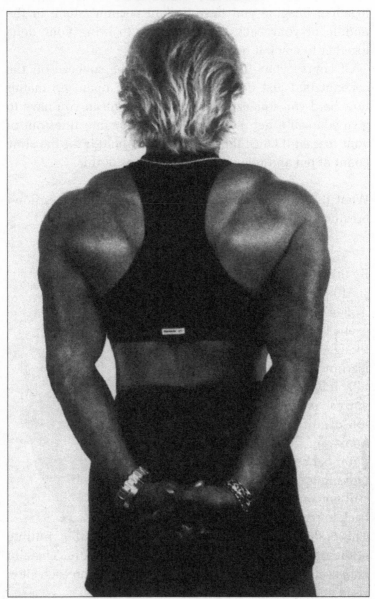

Turn to page 54 and pinpoint the position between 6 and 7 on the diagram. This is the area you're going to hit. Clasp your hands together, as in the photo opposite. Stand tall to straighten out your back. You might hear a few creaks and pops coming from your back but don't worry: it's quite normal. As you stand tall, start to push your right hand down with your left hand. This is the point where I want you to feel it hit. If you can feel it in your shoulders then slacken off the shoulder area. In time you will be able to isolate the area you mean to hit. Give me ten of these on each side. Hold and squeeze for a slow ten count.

SOLITARY SEVENTEEN

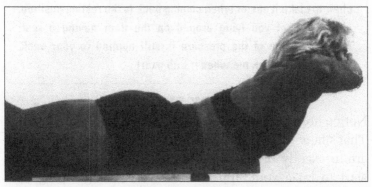

Hold the position above for a slow count of ten. Maybe you won't have the energy to get this far, but assuming the position and contracting the back will start the blood flowing to those underused areas. Some of you might find the position uncomfortable. If so, put something soft underneath your loin area. During this exercise the arms are held out to the side. Try raising the elbows as high as you can – it helps give you the lift you need. Do ten of these and at the height of the movement hold for a slow count of ten.

What it does – It gives excellent strength to the lower back. It's important to keep this area strong: the back ties into the abdominal area. Strong abs doesn't mean you'll be saved from back problems, though. When discussing these two groups of muscles, we do not separate them because they function together to provide stability for the body. You can exercise them separately, but they function together.

TIPS

If you've got a partner who doesn't mind massaging your back, then ask them nicely. Me, I get a towel and use it as if though I was drying my back. Get it glowing red and you will benefit from good blood circulation. Rest your torso on a table or chair to make it easier when coming back to the resting position.

I don't want you lying around on the floor having a rest! This way some of the pressure is still applied to your back. You're gonna thank me when it's all over!

SOLITARY EIGHTEEN

Notice how Storm's back is straight in the photo opposite. That's how your back should be. Use a mirror to check you are in exactly the same pose as above. From this position start to raise your upper torso while still grasping your thigh with both hands. Imagine you have a giant coconut sitting in the middle of your back and the coconut is pressing down on it – your job is to stop it. Feel the tension within your back and keep the squeeze on for a slow count of ten. Do ten reps, alternating between holding the right and left thighs.

When all those muscles start to develop you're gonna thank me for this. Within a few short weeks of applying yourself to this exercise, you're gonna have amazing back strength and not a weight or gym in sight! Although this

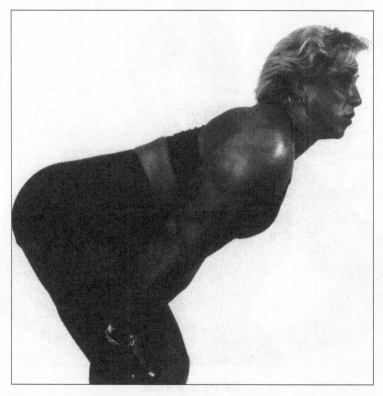

isn't a body part that can be flashed when walking along the high street, at least you'll have the benefit of knowing what's beneath your clothing and this in turn will add a spring to your step.

Hopefully when reproduced in mono the photo above shows the muscle development that all of the previously mentioned exercises relating to the back will give you. Obviously Storm is a professional athlete and to get such development is not yet within your grasp. You may not want such developed muscles, and this is not my aim, but within this book are the ingredients you need to help you attain such definition.

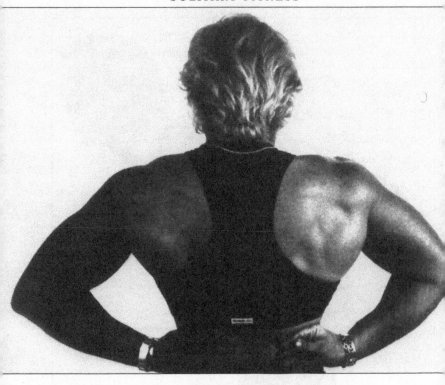

UPPER BACK

The upper back area has seven muscles, which have two functions:
1. To stabilise the scapula (shoulder blade)
2. To move the scapula.

The functions and names of six of the upper-back muscles are listed below. All of these muscles primarily accomplish the retraction, protraction, elevation, depression and rotation of the scapula. The two scapulas are located on the posterior thorax, one to each side, and have no attachment to the axial skeleton. As with the stabilisation function of the rotator cuff, these muscles stabilise and move the

scapula. The function of each muscle is listed below:
- Latissimus dorsi – adduction and abduction of the shoulder joint
- Trapeziums – retraction, elevation, depression and upward rotation of the scapula
- Rhomboid major – retraction of the scapula
- Levator scapulae – elevation of the scapula
- Serratus anterior – protraction of the scapula
- Teres major – adduction, extension and medial rotation of the shoulder joint.

LOWER BACK

The final region of the back to outline is the lower torso. This area consists of the lower back and abdominal area muscles. When discussing these two groups, we do not separate them because together they function to provide stability for the body. You can exercise them separately, but they function together. It is important to spend some good time training the torso region. Outside of aesthetics, the torso is primary to the function of many upper body movements in terms of stability and posture or alignment. These are the muscles of the lower back:
- Psoas major – runs from the lumbar spine through the groin on either side
- Psoas minor – similar action as above but often absent
- Quadratus lumborum – square or rectangular muscle in the back
- Erector spinae – helps keep the spine erect.

SOLITARY ABS

These are gonna blow you away, in more ways than one, ha, ha! Your abdominal muscles are very, very important. They're not there for flashing off by showing a six-pack, they're there to help ward off all sorts of diseases. If, in the end, you develop a six-pack then that's just a spin-off benefit. My real aim here is to get your whole system primed and ready to go. You'll be well aware of the normal sit-ups and crunches, that's fine and we don't want to fully forget them, but here I have the answers to many of your problems.

I don't believe there's an exercise where the abdominal muscles are not used. Just standing around uses them, as does turning in bed and the ability to take a good punch in the guts is one of importance. Does anyone remember the Great Houdini? He was an escapologist. One of his party pieces was to allow you to punch him in the guts while he stood there smiling. One day he asked a young geezer to punch him. BANG! Before Houdini had a chance to flex his abdominal muscles he was hit. He knew something was wrong but he went on with his act. Eventually, after being taken to hospital, he died of peritonitis. As a result of being punched, his internals had been ruptured. Let that be a lesson: expect the unexpected. There was Houdini in all his greatness and for all of his abdominal strength he still ended up dead.

Now don't get me wrong. I'm not saying you want to end up with powerful abdominal muscles so you can go round to your nearest pub on a Saturday night and ask the hardest of the hard to punch you in the guts! But, for the sake of your own vanity, you have to look after the old paunch and tighten it up. You women out there who've had babies will know what I mean. You've tightened up your pelvic floor muscles by sliding around on your rear end, so why not tighten your belly, too?

SOLITARY NINETEEN

Get an old cloth, a piece of paper or a worn-out sock. Tie it to a piece of string or strong thread; anything you've got handy. Hang it so it's just above your head. Fill your lungs up with plenty of air, tilt your head back and make that object move. Be careful you don't initially get a blackout or end up seeing black dots, or even fainting from doing this. It's quite normal for those with weak abs and lungs to keel over like a dead fly. Of course, you've had your doctor give you the once-over before you began exercising, so no real problems if you do see the few black dots to start with.

When you blow and you think you've finished blowing, I want you to give me the final effort in emptying your lungs all over this hanging piece of artwork. You're gonna

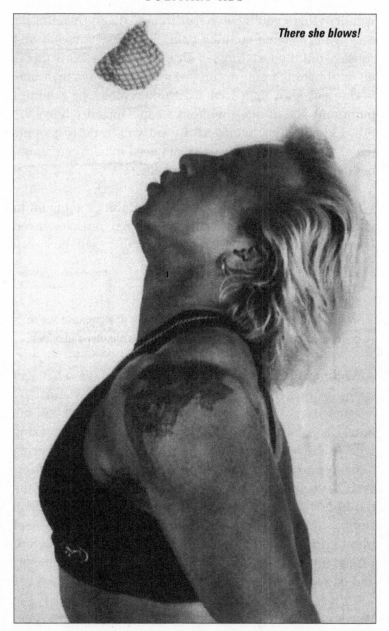

There she blows!

wonder where you'll get the air from to do all this. But it's easy, you're gonna contract your abdominal muscles and squeeze out the last drops of air in your lungs. Now this is no doubt going to blow you away in more ways than one. If you feel faint then have a sit down, don't be a hero. I pump out 100 of these without a gap. Once my lungs are full, I give it some more. All I want you to do is give me ten of them. Rest for as long as you need in between blows, but eventually I want ten off the belt.

What it does – You will feel all sorts of things going on in your throat, chest, lungs and abdominal muscles, even your back will tingle, but primarily this will give you abdominal strength.

> **TIPS**
> **I want you to remember this feeling in your abs because we're going to be doing quite a bit of blowing in this chapter and others.**

Anyone heard of yoga? 'Course you have, it's what you keep in the fridge! I've developed some exercises I learned from an old yogi many years ago. Don't ask me how I became involved with this guy, but it's amazing who you meet behind bars. Ever since, I've been carrying out these exercises. You might think yoga is for softies. Well, I can tell you the guy who taught me was one of the top in his game. He had some connection to one of them Divine Light Missions, but some money problems sent him to prison when a few million quid was embezzled. It turned out he'd done nothing more than sign the cheques and ended up serving time for the real villains.

Word of warning: Yoga is a very specialised way to

maintain your levels of fitness. If you do decide to branch off, then make sure your instructor has at least five years of being a yoga teacher. Anything less than that and you could be asking for trouble.

AORTAL DEATH

The aorta is the main artery of the body that supplies oxygenated blood to the circulatory system. It passes over the heart from the left ventricle and runs down in front of the backbone. I'm gonna give you a big piece of advice here. Call me a know-it-all, call me mad, but what I am about to tell you is fact and will maybe save your life. Believe me when I say that you can die from being too fit!

How old was Churchill when he died? In his nineties! Did he go in for marathon running? Did you see him down the gym jacking up with steroids every week? Did

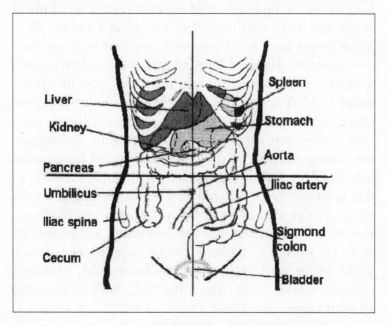

you see him do anything but take things at a steady pace? He slept through the day, puffed on cigars as though they were his life blood and outlived most of his contemporaries, who may well have been a lot fitter than he was. Yet you've got people like Sir Jimmy Saville who's run over 200 marathons and he has had to have open-heart surgery!

If you are too fit then your aorta can become taut. Just falling on your back can rupture the aorta and death is within 30 seconds. Why is it that I read of superfit athletes just dropping down and dying within seconds or men in their forties, who've got themselves into A1 shape, had a full medical and passed with flying colours, who then drop down dead in the best of health? It is my belief that fitness can kill you.

Neither you nor I is going to reach those superfit states because we're applying effort to other things, too. Fitness is not the be-all and end-all of life. Find a hobby, don't make fitness your No. 1 priority ... well, at least not until you've attained a good level of fitness. Now that sounds mad, doesn't it? Me telling you not to get superfit. What I mean is don't spend any more than two hours a day on fitness training. For you, an hour would ideally do, but I guess when you get hooked and those little endorphins start being released by the brain then you're gonna want more! But remember: your reason for attaining fitness is so that you can enjoy a better quality of leisure time doing the things you've always wanted to do. Maybe you've always wanted to own a yacht, but you just didn't feel fit enough to tackle sailing it. Perhaps you're keen to enjoy scenic walks in the countryside, but you haven't felt confident enough to tackle those steep hills. Well, that's what getting fit is all about.

SOLITARY TWENTY

Stand with a slight forward bend of the torso from the waist. Place your palms on your thighs and spread your feet about one metre (three feet) apart. Now tighten the arms, shoulders and neck muscles and lift the ribs.

- Exhale the air from your lungs until every last drop has been pulled out of you. You do this by vigorously contracting the muscles of the abdomen (you've seen how pregnant women get into their breathing routines when going into labour). The chest also gets contracted.

- Press your hands downwards against your thighs as if you were going to pull some air back down into your lungs by raising the ribs, but you're not going to take any air in! Do not allow any air to flow into the lungs ... yet.

- Let the muscles of the abdomen relax to allow your diaphragm to automatically rise up and produce a concave depression of the abdomen. This position has a special yogic name, but since we're not going down Yoga Avenue I don't want to bog you down too much with fancy names.

- Now comes the best part, once all of the breath is out of you I want you to do what you probably last did when you were a kid: push your tummy out fast and immediately pull it in as far as you can, fast. Continue in an out movement until you've just got to take a gasp of air. There are no hard and fast rules on this one coz we all have different capabilities. Count the number of ins and outs and jot it down so that the next time you do it, you'll try to at least equal or beat your record. This is what it's all about, your personal gains!

What it does – Wow, it really helps tone up the digestion system! This exercise massages the abdomen, stimulates the associated nerves, strengthens the muscles and encourages premium health of the abdominal organs. Blood circulation is improved to the whole trunk area and by virtue of this it strengthens all the internal organs. Ever had constipation? It's great for preventing it! Hey, it's also great for diabetes!

TIPS

It's preferable to do this exercise with empty bowels – it's pointless starting and then finding you need to go for a No. 2! Obviously you will not have eaten anything for at least a couple of hours before doing any type of exercise, but this one and most other abdominal exercises are best done early in the day before you start to pump your guts full of food.

SOLITARY TWENTY-ONE

Assume the same position as the previous exercise. Do the following ten times, nice and slow and at your own pace.

- Exhale completely by vigorously contracting the abdominal muscles
- As you do this, simultaneously press your hands against your thighs.
- Hold this condition for as long as it's comfortable
- Slowly release the abdominal muscles and while inhaling return to the upright position.

SOLITARY TWENTY-TWO

For this one you'll need the use of a wall.

- Lie parallel to the ground on your back. Bring your legs on to the wall, keeping them straight, with your trunk inclined at 45 degrees. Try placing a pillow underneath your buttocks if it helps you to get into position to keep your body inclined and properly balanced.

- Get comfortable and completely relaxed.
- Start breathing with the use of your abdomen. As you inhale all that lovely clean air, let your abdomen bulge out. As you exhale, let it sink in.
- The inhalations and exhalations are deliberately slow, rhythmical, continuous and deep.

TIPS

Synchronise inhalation and exhalation with the abdominal movements so there are no jerky movements and it's nice and slow. Make the exhalation longer than the inhalations. Do this for as long as you feel comfortable – usually about ten at a time is enough.

SOLITARY TWENTY-THREE

Assume the same position as the previous exercise. Repeat the following practice for as long as possible.

- Having carried out a few of the breathing movements from the previous exercise, try to isolate the anus.
- Contract the sphincter muscles of the anus for a few seconds without straining. For those who do not know what this is, I would advise you to find out! It's the ring of muscle that gives the final push when you empty your bowels. Imagine it closing the end of a tube leaving your body.
- Relax them for a few seconds.

TIPS

Confine the action to the anal area. The contraction movements, as well as the relaxation of the sphincter muscle, should be performed smoothly and rhythmically. Don't strain! You don't need to synchronise your breathing to the contraction and relaxation of the anus muscles.

SOLITARY TWENTY-FOUR (A)

Assume the same position as the previous exercise. Repeat for as long as you can. While breathing normally, I want you to rapidly contract and relax the sphincter muscles of the anus.

SOLITARY TWENTY-FOUR (B)

Assume the same position as the previous exercise.

- Inhale slowly and deeply while simultaneously contracting the anal sphincter muscles.
- Hold the breath while holding the contraction of the sphincter muscles, too.
- Exhale while simultaneously releasing the contraction of the anus. Perform as many rounds as is comfortably possible.

TIPS

The contraction should be as tight as possible without straining.

There are many more types of these exercises that you can do, but I have shown you the main ones to get you started. I don't want to take you into the world of being able to make your anus muscles contract in a clockwise and an anti-clockwise direction! That's just taking things too far at this early stage within the confines of a little book like this. All the information within this book is sufficient to take you to a platform where you can either stay at the height of fitness or move on to more advanced things. I cannot be the judge of it, only you know the limits you can endure.

You have to be in the frame of mind to want to win fitness. Depression and everyday life can put the block on it and tomorrow, as we know, never comes. So don't fall into that trap of putting things off. Whatever's troubling you, don't dwell on it; just do it! This book will help give you confidence, but confidence has to be a confidence of humility. Don't go round flashing your muscles off to those who wouldn't care less if you're skinny or fat. Save your confidence for yourself and apply it when you need it. Don't use it to put down others less fortunate than yourself. Use it to help those in need of someone like yourself. Your newly found strength can empower the weak and defeat the bully who preys on them. Your whole life can change for the better and when it does I want you to remember how it happened: Solitary Fitness!

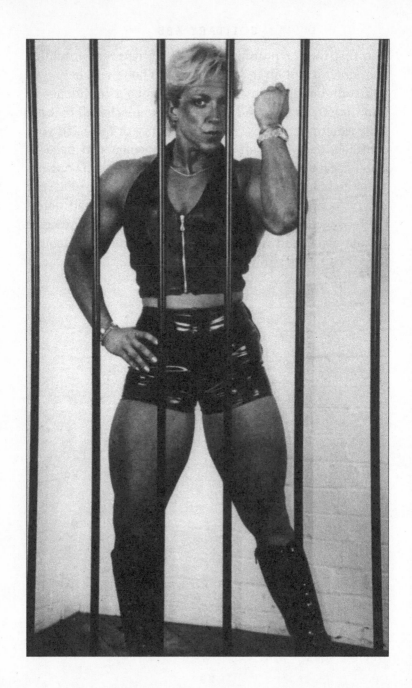

SOLITARY LEGS

The strongest muscle in your body is your tongue, but the biggest muscles are in your legs. The danger is that you can overdevelop those muscles and once overdone they can be a pain to work with. Of course there's nothing worse than the gym freak that pumps out dozens and dozens of bench presses. They've got this massive chest with little spindly legs, ha, ha! At this stage I don't want to go into too much jargon and talk about muscles as if I was a doctor or professor of anatomy coz I'm not! So long as you know where the main muscles are, that's all that counts at this stage. You don't need to know too much about complicated names that will only add to the headache of trying to do the actual exercise in strict form. Look after your legs and they'll give you years of good service. Neglect them and they'll let you down.

For every action there is an equal and opposite reaction. What you put in, you also take out. Your muscles need

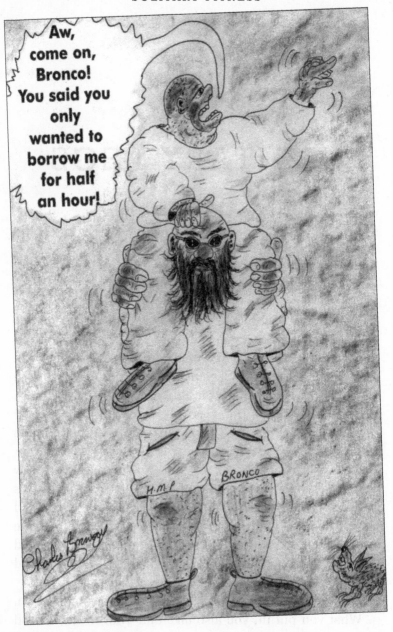

food and oxygen, but a bi-product, known as lactic acid produced within the muscle, has to go someplace. Lactic acid gives your muscle the pain the following morning after you've done some exercises or gardening on the previous day. Ever been on a country walk up steep hills and the following day found that your leg muscles are giving you hell? That's lactic acid at work. I'll give you a tip, bicarbonate of soda helps get rid of this pain. Mix a teaspoonful into a glass of water and knock it back. It takes a little while to work, but it does work.

This little beauty is the calf. When you see a cyclist pedalling along, take a look at their calf muscle. A quality calf muscle is always in the shape of a diamond, and diamonds are a girl's best friend! The leg muscles (hamstrings) tie into the lower back and abdominal muscles (quadriceps) so it's obvious that these muscles are important enough to keep in good shape. There are hundreds of different leg exercises to pick from and for every type of leg exercise there is an expert to guide you, but forget them! The leg exercises in this book are the ones you will use. Maybe in time you can advance to the more flashy ballet moves, but for now stick to them.

Look how ballet dancers move around – such speed, grace and power! They don't go to the gym and squat with 1,000 pounds on their backs, yet they can spring like a

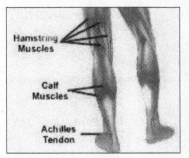
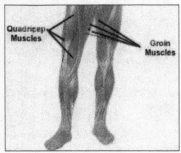

Reebok deer, power a weight up like a gorilla and move like a cheetah! I'm not saying you should take up ballet, but what I am saying is that you don't need to aspire to lifting massive weights to build muscle and define the shape of your legs. The way to fitness is to understand how your body works. I don't mean you need to become a doctor, but what you have to understand is how the parts of your body react when you hit them with a workout. The library is full of books on anatomy, so study one and learn.

Stretching is a way to add dimension to your muscles. Keep working on the muscles with different ideas based on what I've been able to pass on to you. This book is the toolbox!

SOLITARY TWENTY-FIVE

Well, it looks simple enough! Stand in the position shown opposite. Some of you will find standing on one leg

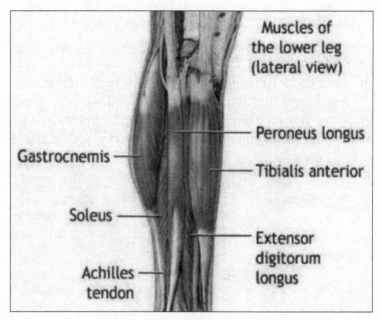

Muscles of the lower leg (lateral view)

Peroneus longus

Tibialis anterior

Gastrocnemis

Soleus

Extensor digitorum longus

Achilles tendon

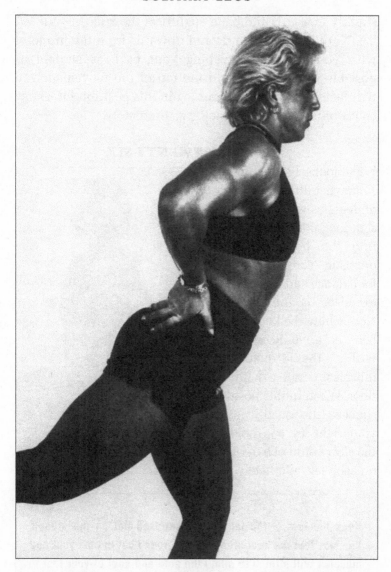

difficult so hold on to a chair if you can't balance properly. Don't worry, the balance part will eventually come naturally to you. Note the position of the hands, lean slightly forwards and bend slightly at the knee of your left leg. Now push backwards and upwards from the hip joint with your right leg, keeping your back as straight as possible. When you get to the top of the movement you will feel the burn. Keep your leg in this position for a slow count of ten. Do ten on each leg, alternately.

SOLITARY TWENTY-SIX

What looks like a lunge is somewhat different in terms of leg positions. From the standing position go down into the position shown opposite. The trailing leg is for balance and the leg being exercised is the right leg. Notice how the knee joint is bent at a 90-degree angle with the quadriceps muscles parallel with the floor. When in this position, squeeze the quadriceps in your right leg and hold for the slow count of ten. Do ten on each leg, alternately.

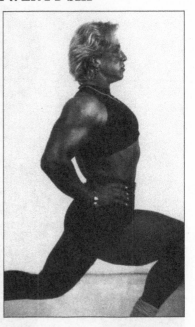

TIP

Keep the foot of the leg being exercised flat on the ground. You may feel the heel lifting off the ground but in time your calf muscles will stretch to allow the sole and heel of your foot to remain in contact with the floor throughout.

SOLITARY TWENTY-SEVEN

Assume the position as below. Keeping your back as straight as possible, raise your right leg from the hip. When you get to the top of the movement you will feel the burn. Keep the leg in this position for a slow count of ten. Do ten on each leg, alternately.

SOLITARY TWENTY-EIGHT

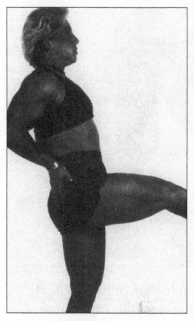

This exercise partially exercises the lower-back muscles while working the hamstring, too. Lift your right leg as close to you as possible – you should feel the hamstring start to burn. Try to isolate this feeling and squeeze the hamstring. Keep the leg in this position for a slow count of ten. Do ten on each leg, alternately.

Leg muscles
• Quadriceps – A group of muscles lying on the front of the thigh, their function is to straighten the leg through the extension of the knee joint.
• Hip Flexors Illiopsoas – Two muscles that connect part of the lower spine and hipbone to the top of the thigh. Their function is to lift the leg to the front (flexion of the hip joint).
• Adductors – A group of muscles lying on the inside of the thigh, their function is to move the leg towards

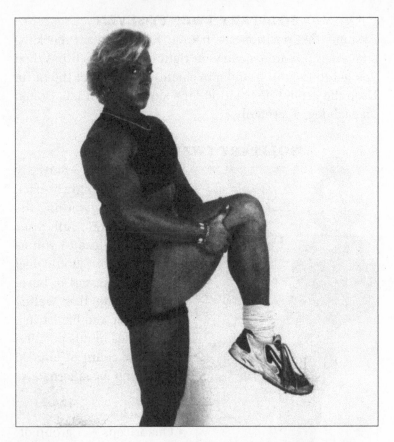

the mid-line of the body (adduction of the hip joint).

- Hamstrings – A group of muscles lying on the rear of the thigh. Their function is to move the leg towards the mid-line of the body (adduction of the hip joint).
- Gastrocnemius & Soleus – Two muscles lying to the rear of the lower leg, their function is to point the foot downwards (plantarflexion of the ankle joint).
- Tibialis Anterior – A muscle lying mainly on the front of the lower leg, its function is to point the foot upwards (dorsiflexion of the ankle joint).

SOLITARY NECK

You've either been blessed with a swanlike neck or it's gone flabby! Men and women alike spend fortunes on neck-firming potions that promise the impossible. Look, if these creams worked, then plastic surgeons would go bust! There's no instant fix for a saggy neck. However, there is a way to give the neck a makeover that will cost you next to nothing. You're gonna make your own neck-firming potion, but more of this later on!

Through your neck run some very important pieces of pipe work – your spinal cord, arteries and your windpipe. There is also a very small bone located near to the front of the neck; if it gets broken then it can result in instantaneous death. The SAS like to do a straight-fingered jab to this area, and now you know why. I'm not saying that these exercises will prevent an SAS attack from killing you, but they will certainly improve that saggy look.

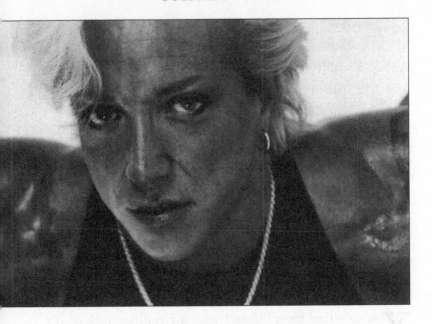

SOLITARY TWENTY-NINE

Get two bowls or two pans or anything that will hold water.
Fill one of the vessels with fresh cold water, about 2 litres
(31/2 pints) and chuck a couple of spoonfuls of salt in with
it. Place the vessels next to each other and now suck a
mouthful of water up from the full vessel, holding it in
your mouth. Move your head over to the empty vessel and
spit it out. Don't let the water run out of your mouth,
forcibly spit it out.

When you've shifted about a litre (13/4 pints) of the
stuff, stop. The reason for putting salt in with the water is
that it acts as a natural cleansing agent for your gums and
is also good for clearing up ulcers in the mouth. This
should also get your muscles working. Don't expect to do
this in a few mouthfuls: in time you'll become very
competent and able to up the amount of water you use.

SOLITARY THIRTY

Two exercises in one: first, assume the position as in the illustration. For those with a stiff back, it might be best if you go as far back as you feel comfortable with. When in the position shown, or near enough to it, rest your chin on your chest and then return to the position shown. Hold for a count of ten.

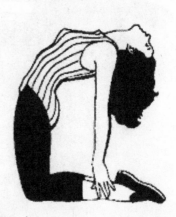

Do ten of these. Make sure the movement is nice and slow – we don't want any strains, do we? As well as toning up your neck, this also gives your back a nice stretch.

TIPS

When in the position shown, open and close your mouth as wide as possible. In time increase the reps.

SOLITARY THIRTY-ONE

Get a pillow, place it under your chin and tilt your head forward to grip the pillow between your chin and chest. Now gently tug at the pillow with your hands as if to pull it out, but you're going to resist this by gripping it even more tightly by pressing down with your chin. Hold for a slow count of ten. Do ten of these.

SOLITARY THIRTY-TWO

Holding your hand on your forehead, push against it with your head. When you reach the point of most resistance, hold for a slow count of ten. Do ten of these.

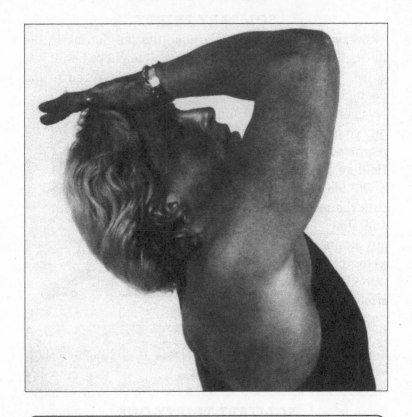

SOLITARY THIRTY-THREE

Anyone for tennis? Have you a spare tennis ball lying about the place? Anything similar will do: a rolled-up sock, for instance. Get down on all fours, like a dog. Find a space with about 1.8m (6ft) of clear runway in front of you. Now, with your chin, start rolling the ball along the floor. In time, find a larger area. Imagine me in my cage doing this!

> **TIP**
> Now you lot are gonna have shag pile carpet on the floors of your mansion; me, I've got cold concrete! Don't do it on the shag pile coz you'll get friction burns on your knees! The aim is to roll the ball, not push it.

SOLITARY THIRTY-FOUR

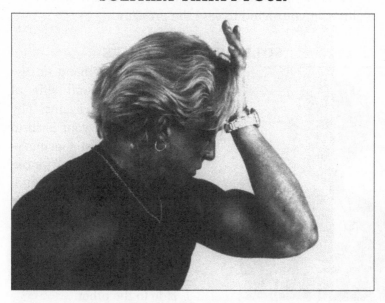

Holding your hand on your forehead, push against it with your head. Resist the movement by applying more pressure from your hand.

This is not the same exercise as Solitary Thirty-two. Note the difference in your head position, slightly off-centre and looking slightly to the side. When you reach the point of most resistance, hold for a slow count of ten.

Do ten of these with each hand, alternately changing your head position to face the side of the pushing arm.

> **TIP**
> Keep your back straight; don't hold your breath or you're likely to have a blackout! Don't do this exercise with oily hands or you might slip. Avoid clenching your teeth together as this can loosen dental fillings

Those of you with delicate skin might find it best to use a glove on your hand to ease the pressure.

SOLITARY THIRTY-FIVE

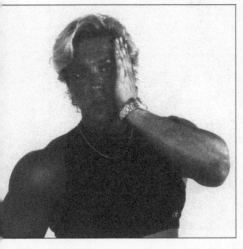

Holding your hand on the temple area and side of your face, push against it by trying to turn your head to the side. Resist the movement by applying more pressure from your hand. When you reach the point of most resistance, hold for a slow count of ten.

Do ten of these on each side, alternating from one side to the other.

SOLITARY THIRTY-SIX

Find a suitably solid place to press upwards against with a pillow placed on top of your head. Anything you can use to apply a downward pressure will do. For example, stand on some boxes beneath the frame of a door, while pressing the pillow to the underside of the frame. Only apply slight pressure to keep the pillow in place. Now comes the part where you keep your head still but move your body from the neck down in very small circles! Do ten clockwise and then another ten anti-clockwise.

SOLITARY THIRTY-SEVEN

Holding your hand on the side of your head, push against it with your head. Resist the movement by applying more pressure from your hand. When you reach the point of most resistance, hold for a slow count of ten. Do ten of these on each side.

I have deliberately omitted certain exercises from this book because I feel they may be too dangerous for the beginner. Maybe if I do a follow-up *Solitary Fitness* book I'll include them, but, in the meantime, crack on!

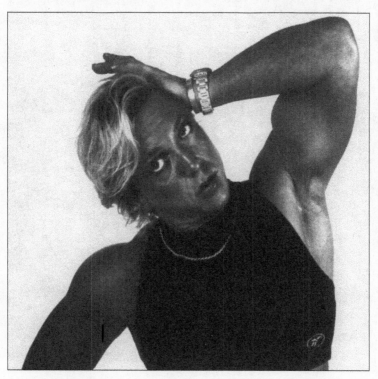

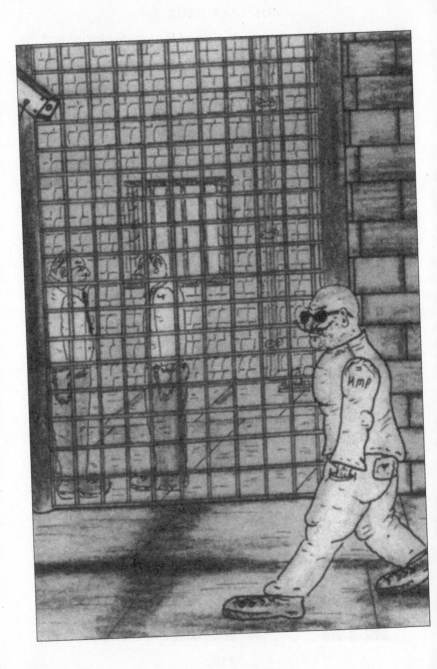

SOLITARY WAY

I am the way; I am the light ... said Bronson! Follow me, my way, the Solitary Way. This is the chapter that's gonna be your toolkit to fix your body. I've devised the workouts for optimum efficiency. Don't just follow the routines I've listed: you have to aid and abet the workouts in conjunction with the other Solitary chapters. What follows is a 32-day routine.

Don't think you can follow the workouts listed in a robotic fashion. If you just want to get through the routines, then fine, be my guest ... but don't go telling people you used my workouts coz they're gonna laugh at me. Follow my instructions to the letter and put some effort into the overall programme! Study my way until you know it back to front. Don't be frightened to experiment – how do you think I discovered the best way to become fit and fast? I haven't applied myself to this book just for the fun of it: it's your turn now!

SOLITARY DAY ONE

Always start out by warming up and stretching. Do this religiously and don't skip it, no matter what. Vary the warm-up so you don't become bored. Even if you're pushed for time, don't do the routine without doing the warm-up and stretching first. *Find* the time.

Some of you might find the following very tiring. If so, cut the number to do in half. Do your best, but don't kill yourself and always remember: Sunday is a day of rest!

1.	Normal press-ups	1 x 10
2.	Sit-ups	1 x 10
3.	Squats	1 x 10
4.	Squat-thrusts	1 x 10
5.	Burpees	1 x 10
6.	Star jumps	1 x 10
7.	Step-ups	1 x 10
8.	Solitary Nine	Do the same amount as in the chapter
9.	Solitary Eleven	Do the same amount as in the chapter
10.	Normal press-ups	Do the same amount as in the chapter
11.	Solitary Two	Do the same amount as in the chapter

SOLITARY DAY TWO

1.	Solitary One	Do the same amount as in the chapter
2.	Normal press-ups	1 x 10
3.	Solitary Three	Do the same amount as in the chapter
4.	Solitary Two	Do the same amount as in the chapter
5.	Solitary Five	Do the same amount as in the chapter
6.	Solitary Seven	Do the same amount as in the chapter
7.	Squat-thrusts	1 x 10
8.	Star jumps	1 x 10

SOLITARY DAY THREE

1. Solitary One   Do the same amount as in the chapter
2. Solitary Two   Do the same amount as in the chapter
3. Solitary Six   Do the same amount as in the chapter
4. Solitary Seven   Do the same amount as in the chapter
5. Burpees   1 x 10
6. Star jumps   1 x 10
7. Solitary Eight   Do the same amount as in the chapter
8. Solitary Eleven   Do the same amount as in the chapter
9. Solitary Eighteen   Do the same amount as in the chapter

SOLITARY DAY FOUR

1. Squat-thrusts   1 x 10
2. Solitary Seventeen   Do the same amount as in the chapter
3. Solitary Thirteen   Do the same amount as in the chapter
4. Solitary Eighteen   Do the same amount as in the chapter
5. Star jumps   1 x 10
6. Solitary Stretch   Page 20 x 10
7. Solitary Stretch   Page 21 x 10
8. Squat-thrusts   1 x 10

SOLITARY DAY FIVE

1. Solitary Two   Do the same amount as in the chapter
2. Solitary Three   Do the same amount as in the chapter
3. Solitary Four   Do the same amount as in the chapter
4. Solitary Ten   Do the same amount as in the chapter
5. Solitary Eleven   Do the same amount as in the chapter
6. Solitary One   Do the same amount as in the chapter
7. Solitary Thirteen   Do the same amount as in the chapter
8. Solitary Sixteen   Do the same amount as in the chapter
9. Burpees   1 x 10
10. Squat-thrusts   1 x 10

SOLITARY DAY SIX

1.	Solitary Thirteen	Do the same amount as in the chapter
2.	Solitary Fourteen	Do the same amount as in the chapter
3.	Solitary Fifteen	Do the same amount as in the chapter
4.	Solitary Sixteen	Do the same amount as in the chapter
5.	Solitary Seventeen	Do the same amount as in the chapter
6.	Solitary Eighteen	Do the same amount as in the chapter
7.	Solitary One	Do the same amount as in the chapter
8.	Squat-thrusts	1 x 10
9.	Sit-ups	1 x 10
10.	Solitary Nineteen	Do the same amount as in the chapter
11.	Solitary Twenty	Do the same amount as in the chapter

SOLITARY DAY SEVEN

1.	Step-ups	1 x 10
2.	Solitary Twenty-eight	Do the same amount as in the chapter
3.	Squat-thrusts	1 x 10
4.	Solitary Twenty-six	1 x 10
5.	Star jumps	2 sets x 10 reps
6.	Squats	2 x 10
7.	Solitary Twenty-six	1 x 10

SOLITARY DAY EIGHT

1.	Solitary Thirty	Do the same amount as in the chapter
2.	Solitary Thirty-one	Do the same amount as in the chapter
3.	Solitary Thirty-two	Do the same amount as in the chapter
4.	Solitary Thirty-four	Do the same amount as in the chapter
5.	Solitary Thirty-five	Do the same amount as in the chapter
6.	Solitary Thirty-seven	Do the same amount as in the chapter
7.	Solitary Fourteen	Do the same amount as in the chapter
8.	Solitary Fifteen	Do the same amount as in the chapter
9.	Solitary Sixteen	Do the same amount as in the chapter
10.	Solitary Seventeen	Do the same amount as in the chapter

11. Solitary Stretch   Page xx, 1 x 10 reps

12. Solitary Twenty-eight Do the same amount as in the chapter

13. Solitary Twenty-seven Do the same amount as in the chapter

14. Squat-thrusts   1 x 10

15. Solitary Twenty-five   Do the same amount as in the chapter

16. Burpees   1 x 10

SOLITARY DAY NINE

1. Solitary Nineteen   Do the same amount as in the chapter

2. Sit-ups   2 x 10

3. Solitary Twenty   Do the same amount as in the chapter

4. Solitary Twenty-one   Do the same amount as in the chapter

5. Solitary Twenty-two   Do the same amount as in the chapter

6. Sit-ups   3 x 10

SOLITARY DAY TEN

1. Leg Stretch (page xx) 1 x 10 (each leg)

2. Squats   2 x 10

3. Solitary Twenty-six   2 x 10 (each leg)

4. Solitary Twenty-five   2 x 10 (each leg)

5. Solitary Twenty-eight 2 x 10 (each leg)

6. Star jumps   2 x 10

7. Squat-thrusts   2 x 10

8. Leg Stretch (page xx) 2 x 10 (each leg)

SOLITARY DAY ELEVEN

1. Solitary Thirty   Do the same amount as in the chapter

2. Solitary Thirty-one   Do the same amount as in the chapter

3. Solitary Seventeen   Do the same amount as in the chapter

4. Solitary Stretch   Page 21, 1 x 10

5. Solitary Eighteen   Do the same amount as in the chapter

6. Solitary Fourteen   Do the same amount as in the chapter

7. Solitary Six   Do the same amount as in the chapter

8.	Solitary Seven	Do the same amount as in the chapter
9.	Solitary Nine	Do the same amount as in the chapter
10.	Solitary Eight	Do the same amount as in the chapter
11.	Press-ups	1 x 10
12.	Solitary One	Do the same amount as in the chapter
13.	Solitary Thirteen	Do the same amount as in the chapter
14.	Solitary Stretch	Page 20, 1 x 10
15.	Squat-thrusts	1 x 10
16.	Burpees	1 x 10

SOLITARY DAY TWELVE

1.	Solitary Two	Do the same amount as in the chapter
2.	Solitary Three	Do the same amount as in the chapter
3.	Solitary Four	Do the same amount as in the chapter
4.	Solitary Five	Do the same amount as in the chapter
5.	Solitary Ten	Do the same amount as in the chapter
6.	Solitary Eleven	Do the same amount as in the chapter
8.	Solitary Twelve	Do the same amount as in the chapter

SOLITARY DAY THIRTEEN

1.	Solitary Nineteen	x 20
2.	Solitary Twenty	Beat your record
3.	Solitary Twenty-one	Do the same amount as in the chapter
4.	Solitary Twenty-three	Do the same amount as in the chapter
5.	Solitary Twenty-four	Do the same amount as in the chapter
6.	Sit-ups	3 x 20
7.	Solitary Stretch	Page 20, 1 x 20
8.	Solitary Stretch	Page 21, 2 x 10
9.	Solitary Seventeen	2 x 10

SOLITARY DAY FOURTEEN

1.	Solitary Twenty-five	Do the same amount as in the chapter
2.	Solitary Twenty-six	Do the same amount as in the chapter

3.	Solitary Twenty-seven	Do the same amount as in the chapter
4.	Solitary Twenty-eight	Do the same amount as in the chapter
5.	Step-ups	2 x 10
6.	Squats	3 x 10
7.	Star jumps	2 x 10
8.	Burpees	2 x 10
9.	Squat-thrusts	1 x 10
10.	Squats	2 x 5
11.	Star jumps	1 x 5
12.	Squats	1 x 5
13.	Step-ups	1 x 10
14.	Burpees	1 x 5
15.	Squats	1 x 5
17.	Solitary Stretch	Page 18, 2 x 5

SOLITARY DAY FIFTEEN

1.	Solitary Thirty-seven	Do the same amount as in the chapter
2.	Solitary Thirty-six	Do the same amount as in the chapter
3.	Solitary Thirty-five	Do the same amount as in the chapter
4.	Solitary Thirty-four	Do the same amount as in the chapter
5.	Solitary Thirty-three	Do the same amount as in the chapter
6.	Solitary Thirty-two	Do the same amount as in the chapter
7.	Solitary Thirty	Do the same amount as in the chapter
8.	Solitary One	Double the amount in the chapter
9.	Solitary Two	Double the amount in the chapter
10.	Solitary Three	Double the amount in the chapter
11.	Solitary Four	Double the amount in the chapter
12.	Press-ups	2 x 10
13.	Solitary Four	Do the same amount as in the chapter
14.	Solitary Two	Do the same amount as in the chapter

SOLITARY DAY SIXTEEN

1. Solitary Thirteen   Do the same amount as in the chapter
2. Solitary Fourteen   Do the same amount as in the chapter
3. Solitary Sixteen   Do the same amount as in the chapter
4. Solitary Seventeen   Do the same amount as in the chapter
5. Solitary Five   Do the same amount as in the chapter
6. Solitary Six   Do the same amount as in the chapter
7. Solitary Seven   Do the same amount as in the chapter
8. Solitary Eight   Do the same amount as in the chapter

9. Solitary Nine   Do the same amount as in the chapter
10. Solitary Ten   Do the same amount as in the chapter
11. Solitary Eleven   Do the same amount as in the chapter
12. Solitary Twelve   Do the same amount as in the chapter

SOLITARY DAY SEVENTEEN

1. Solitary Twenty-five   Do the same amount as in the chapter
2. Solitary twenty-six   Do the same amount as in the chapter
3. Solitary Twenty-seven Do the same amount as in the chapter
4. Solitary Twenty-eight Do the same amount as in the chapter
5. Solitary Nineteen   Do the same amount as in the chapter
6. Solitary Twenty   Beat your record
7. Solitary Twenty-one   Do the same amount as in the chapter
8. Solitary Twenty-two   Do the same amount as in the chapter
9. Solitary Twenty-three Do the same amount as in the chapter
10. Solitary Twenty-four
    (a)   Do the same amount as in the chapter
11. Solitary Twenty-four
    (b)   Do the same amount as in the chapter
12. Sit-ups   3 x 10
13. Solitary Twelve   Do the same amount as in the chapter
14. Solitary Eleven   Do the same amount as in the chapter

124

SOLITARY DAY EIGHTEEN

1.	Press-ups	3 x 10
2.	Sit-ups	3 x 10
3.	Squats	1 x 10
4.	Squat-thrusts	1 x 10
5.	Burpees	2 x 10
6.	Star jumps	1 x 10
7.	Press-ups	2 x 10
8.	Sit-ups	2 x 10
9.	Squats	1 x 5
10.	Squat-thrusts	1 x 5
11.	Burpees	2 x 5
12.	Star jumps	1 x 5
13.	Step-ups	1 x 5
14.	Sit-ups	1 x 10
15.	Squats	2 x 5
16.	Squat-thrusts	2 x 5
17.	Burpees	1 x 5
18.	Star jumps	2 x 10
19.	Solitary Stretch	Page 18, 2 x 10

SOLITARY DAY NINETEEN

1.	Solitary Thirty-three	Do the same amount as in the chapter
2.	Solitary Five	Do the same amount as in the chapter
3.	Solitary Four	Do the same amount as in the chapter
4.	Solitary Eleven	Do the same amount as in the chapter
5.	Solitary Thirteen	Do the same amount as in the chapter
6.	Solitary One	Do the same amount as in the chapter
7.	Solitary Nine	Do the same amount as in the chapter
8.	Solitary Eighteen	Do the same amount as in the chapter
9.	Solitary Nineteen	Do the same amount as in the chapter
10.	Solitary Twenty	Do the same amount as in the chapter
11.	Solitary Twenty-six	Do the same amount as in the chapter

SOLITARY DAY TWENTY

1. Solitary Stretch   Page 20, 2 x 10
2. Solitary Stretch   Page 21, 2 x 10
3. Solitary Stretch   Page 18, 2 x 10 (each leg)
4. Solitary Twenty-eight 2 x 10 (each leg)
5. Solitary Eighteen   2 x 10
6. Solitary Thirteen   2 x 10

SOLITARY DAY TWENTY-ONE

1. Solitary Twenty-eight Do the same amount as in the chapter
2. Solitary Twenty-seven Do the same amount as in the chapter
3. Solitary Twenty-six   Do the same amount as in the chapter
4. Solitary Twenty-five Do the same amount as in the chapter
5. Star jumps   2 x 10
6. Sit-ups   3 x 10
7. Solitary Twenty   Beat your record
8. Solitary Twenty-one Do the same amount as in the chapter
9. Solitary Twelve   Do the same amount as in the chapter
10. Solitary Fourteen   Do the same amount as in the chapter
11. Solitary Sixteen   Do the same amount as in the chapter
12. Solitary Nine   Do the same amount as in the chapter
13. Solitary One   Do the same amount as in the chapter
14. Solitary Twenty-nine   2 litres (31/2 pints)
15. Solitary Thirty-three   12 metres (40 feet)
16. Solitary Four   Do the same amount as in the chapter
17. Solitary Two   Do the same amount as in the chapter
18. Solitary Ten   Do the same amount as in the chapter
19. Solitary Eleven   Do the same amount as in the chapter
20. Solitary Stretch   Page 20, 2 x 10
21. Solitary Stretch   Page 21, 2 x 10
22. Solitary Stretch   Page 18, 2 x 10 (each leg)
23. Solitary Twenty-eight 2 x 10 (each leg)
24. Solitary Eighteen   2 x 10

25. Solitary Thirteen   2 x 10

SOLITARY DAY TWENTY-TWO

1.	Press-ups	4 x 10
2.	Solitary Eleven	4 x 10
3.	Press-ups	3 x 10
4.	Solitary Eleven	3 x 10
5.	Press-ups	2 x 10
6.	Solitary Eleven	2 x 10
7.	Press-ups	1 x 10
8.	Solitary Eleven	1 x 10
9.	Solitary Four	3 x 10 (each arm)
10.	Solitary Three	3 x 10 (each arm)
11.	Solitary Four	2 x 10 (each arm)
12.	Solitary Three	2 x 10 (each arm)
13.	Solitary Four	1 x 10 (each arm)
14.	Solitary Three	1 x 10 (each arm)
15.	Press-ups	To exhaustion

SOLITARY DAY TWENTY-THREE

1.	Sit-ups	1 x 20
2.	Solitary Twenty	Beat record
3.	Sit-ups	2 x 15
4.		Solitary Twenty Beat record
5.	Sit-ups	3 x 10
6.	Solitary Twenty	Beat record
7.	Sit-ups	4 x 10
8.	Solitary Twenty	Beat record
9.	Sit-ups	To exhaustion
10.	Solitary Twenty	Beat record
11.	Solitary Eighteen	1 x 10
12.	Solitary Seventeen	1 x 10
13.	Solitary Eighteen	1 x 15

14. Solitary Seventeen   To exhaustion
15. Star jumps   To exhaustion

SOLITARY DAY TWENTY-FOUR

1. Solitary Six   1 x 10 (each side)
2. Solitary One   10 of each
3. Press-ups   1 x 10
4. Solitary Six   2 x 10 (each side)
5. Solitary One   15 of each
6. Press-ups   2 x 10
7. Solitary Six   3 x 10 (each side)
8. Solitary One   20 of each
9. Press-ups   3 x 10
10. Solitary Six   To exhaustion
11. Solitary One   To exhaustion
12. Press-ups   To exhaustion

SOLITARY DAY TWENTY-FIVE

1. Solitary Thirteen   1 x 10
2. Solitary Fifteen   10 (each side)
3. Solitary Thirteen   2 x 10
4. Solitary Fifteen   12 (each side)
5. Solitary Thirteen   2 x 12
6. Solitary Fifteen   15 (each side)
7. Solitary Thirteen   2 x 15
8. Solitary Fifteen   20 (each side)
9. Press-ups   To exhaustion
10. Solitary Sixteen   10 (each side)
11. Solitary Seventeen   1 x 10
12. Solitary Sixteen   12 (each side)
13. Solitary Seventeen   2 x 12
14. Solitary Sixteen   15 (each side)
15. Solitary Seventeen   2 x 15

16. Press-ups   To exhaustion

SOLITARY DAY TWENTY-SIX

1. Solitary Thirty-one   1 x 10
2. Solitary Twenty-nine Do the same amount as in the chapter
3. Solitary Thirty   1 x 10
4. Solitary Thirty-two   1 x 10
5. Solitary Thirty-six   10 (each way)
6. Solitary Thirty-one   1 x 15
7. Solitary Twenty-nine 3 litres (51/4 pints)
8. Solitary Thirty   2 x 10
9. Solitary Thirty-two   2 x 10
10. Solitary Thirty-six   5 (each way)

SOLITARY DAY TWENTY-SEVEN

1. Solitary Twenty-six   10 (each leg)
2. Solitary Twenty-seven 10 (each leg)
3. Star jumps   1 x 10
4. Squats   1 x 10
5. Solitary Twenty-six   12 (each leg)
6. Solitary Twenty-seven 12 (each leg)
7. Star jumps   1 x 12
8. Squats   1 x 12
9. Solitary Twenty-six   15 (each leg)
10. Solitary Twenty-seven 15 (each leg)
11. Star jumps   1 x 15
12. Squats   1 x 50
13. Solitary Twenty-six   To exhaustion
14. Solitary Twenty-seven To exhaustion
15. Star jumps   To exhaustion
16. Squats   To exhaustion
17. Solitary Twenty-eight 10 (each leg)

SOLITARY DAY TWENTY-EIGHT

Press-ups advanced – Walk up and down, then do ten press-ups and get back on your feet. Walk up and down, and do nine, and so on, back down to one. Then back up to one, two, three, etc. Add it up. Would you believe, that's 110! Increase the starting amount by one every day and in a year ... well, let's not rush it, just enjoy what you do.

You wait till you're pushing press-ups in their tons! You wait till you feel the flow in your body and the lightness in your head. I'm giving you something here that money can't buy: total and utter supreme fitness beyond your expectations! I actually do a lot more exercises, but those listed in this chapter are my main ones, which I recommend you to start with.

Now you need to set yourself a goal. I'll leave that to you, as we are all different. Some of you will do sets of 50, others sets of ten – it doesn't matter, it's what feels best for you. I'd say, start off with tens; do ten of them all, time it and then do ten sets, so that's 100 of each exercise. Do it every day, Monday to Saturday, and remember Sunday is a rest day. After a month, up each set to 15, and so on. Have faith in it, as it will work if you work at it! After a workout you'll feel good, proud of yourself and a better person. Up till now I've saved you money, I've made your life better, I've given you some serious advice and so I'd like some feedback on how it's been for you. How do you see it? How do you feel? Has it worked for you, etc.? I'd be intrigued to know.

This must have been a bad day for me coz normally I smash out 131 press-ups in 60 seconds! Records are there for breaking. Me, I would like to see you reach your own level. Forget about records like mine, give some thought

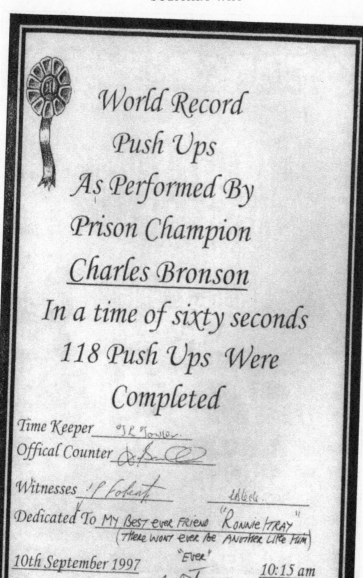

World Record
Push Ups
As Performed By
Prison Champion
<u>Charles Bronson</u>
In a time of sixty seconds
118 Push Ups Were
Completed

Time Keeper _J L Towler._

Offical Counter _____

Witnesses _J P Foley_   _lablede._

Dedicated To MY BEST ever FRIEND "RONNIE KRAY"
(THERE WONT ever be ANoTHER LIKE HIM)

<u>10th September 1997</u>   "Ever"   <u>10:15 am</u>

Charles Bronson

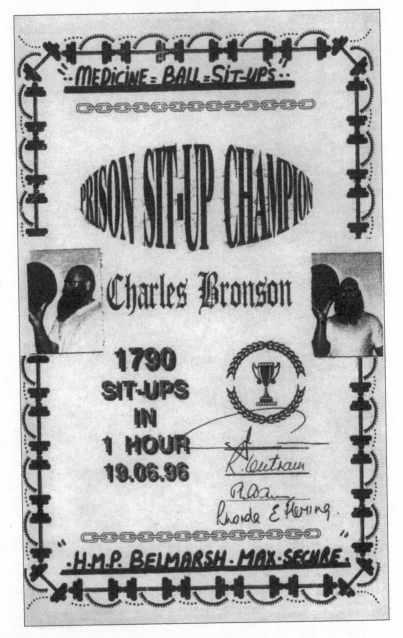

to how you can best improve and strive to achieve it. When you attain your goal, whatever it is, then you can feel satisfied that you did your best – better than breaking any record.

The sit-ups record above was carried out while holding a medicine ball. Hell, what's the use of doing sit-ups without some sort of resistance when you get to my level of fitness? Carry out the sit-ups how I've taught you with a strict eye to correct form. Don't lose correct form. Incorrectly done, a simple exercise like this can damage your spine. My record was achieved using strict form, chest to the ground and elbows just about locked out at the top of the movement, with a rigid back. I've seen my record broken, but with a less than strict style. Sure, you can double this amount or even more if you perform them this way, but always concentrate on strict form.

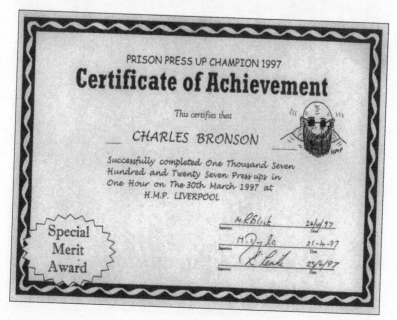

PRISON PRESS UP CHAMPION 1997

Certificate of Achievement

This certifies that

CHARLES BRONSON

Successfully completed One Thousand Seven Hundred and Twenty Seven Press ups in One Hour on The 30th March 1997 at H.M.P. LIVERPOOL

Special Merit Award

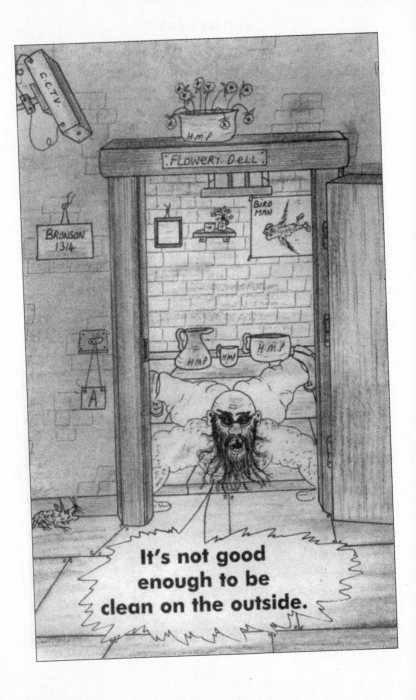

It's not good enough to be clean on the outside.

SOLITARY
CLEANSE

In this chapter I will detail some of the techniques that have worked for me, but I highly recommend consulting a doctor before practising any of them on yourself, as not all of them are common medical practice – it's my way! Be Empty your mind

OK, so you want to know how to stay young and healthy. I suppose I gotta tell you the secret of youth: laughter. You have to find a way to shed all of those inner worries. Why pay a therapist good money when laughter can cleanse you of all that misery within? Yes, laughter keeps the body clear of tension. Half an hour is a good session – laugh so much you cry, your ribs hurt, you sweat, your lungs burn and you laugh to the point of insanity.

Get a copy of 'The Laughing Policeman' song. You know the one they used to play at the seaside fun fair? Start off like that. Soon you'll not need any assistance; you'll be able to do it on your own. Obviously you need to pick the right place to do it as it's madness and you could get locked up! But it's great: it's a relief, a release and it tightens the body tissues, strengthens the muscles of your face and neck and tones up your inner vocal cords. Would you believe that laughing also burns off calories? A good half-hour session and you'll burn right into that fat. Crazy, but fact. So all the guys who used to hear me laughing in the prison dungeons now know why. I hadn't lost the plot, I was actually working out.

I bet that Arnie couldn't tell you this! Could you see any muscle-bound prat laughing? They take it all too serious, see. It's an illness with them freaks! For me it's a pleasure. I'm not after awesome muscle and bulk; I'm after a ripe old age, fitness, health and happiness. No trainer, athlete or anyone else could ever give you such advice, but you got it from me, the Solitary Man! Enjoy it, have a laugh!

very careful when performing any of my techniques.

FASTING

A good tip: every so often, say once a month, go two days without food. But before you do this make sure you have a clean bill of health and consult a doctor. Just drink lots of fluids. I just do water, but you should have fruit juices too – I'd do juices as well if I were outside! Anyway, the reason for this is simple: you need to clean out. Like a motor coated with engine oil, your body needs a clean and there is no better way to do it than fasting. If you can't survive without food, just eat fruit, but, if you can't go two days without eating, you're a weak person.

Yeah, clear out all the filth that lies in your gut and you'll feel lighter, faster and healthier. I also believe that by doing

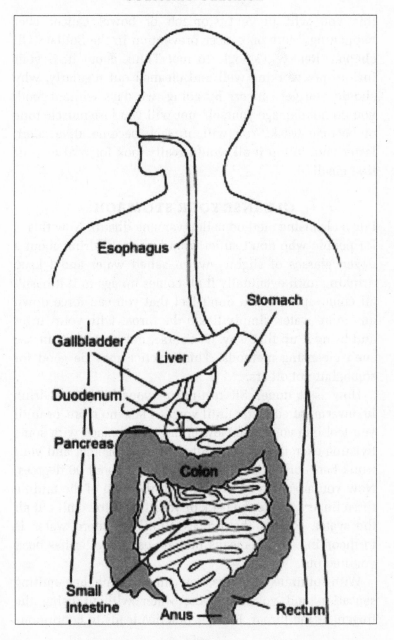

this you will prevent stomach or bowel cancer ever happening. More on cancer prevention in the Solitary Oil chapter. Really, it's logic to me! Think about it: if your insides are working well and cleaned out regularly, why should you get cancer? By going two days without food, you do not damage yourself, nor will you lose muscle tone or become weak. You will, in fact, become alive, alert, faster and, to top it all, you'll really look forward to your first meal!

CLEANSE YOUR STOMACH

I do a cleansing method called vamana-dhauti. Now this is for people who don't suffer from bulimia! I drink about a dozen glasses of slightly warm salted water and I keep drinking until eventually it all comes up again. If it hasn't all come up, and you don't feel that you can force down any more water, simply tickle the throat with your finger and bring it up that way. Of course, not everyone can use such cleansing methods. This practice may be good for some, but not others.

How is it done? Sit resting on your heels and drink lukewarm salted water until you can take no more, or until you feel like vomiting. Now churn the stomach with some twisting exercises. Stand with your feet together and your trunk bent forwards to form an angle of about 90 degrees. Now you are ready to vomit. With the help of the middle three fingers, tickle the back of your throat to vomit out all the water. Repeat the process until no more water is forthcoming, which means that almost all water has been vomited out.

With continued practice, you can stimulate the vomiting sensation and vomit out the water without using the fingers at the throat. Further practice leads to continuous vomiting of all the water through the mouth as if it is coming out like a jet.

AIR CAN BE YOUR FRIEND

Another system I use for cleansing the stomach is called plavini-pranayama. It's where I swallow big mouthfuls of air into my stomach! Have you ever had anyone belch in your face? Stinks, doesn't it? It has a smell all of its own, unique! Along with the air swallowed, I belch out toxic gases.

FLUSH OUT YOUR SINUSES

Ever had a cold? It all starts in the nose. Did you know if they could squirt superheated steam into your nose when you have a cold it would kill the germs of the cold bug? Since doing so wouldn't be very safe, we all have to put up with the common cold – or do we? Sutra Neti is the term given to one of

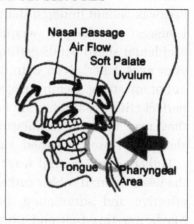

the most powerful and beneficial cleansing methods I've ever used, yet it's one of the most simple, too. I do this soon after rising in conjunction with the rest of my morning cleansing activities.

Inhale a dampened 46cm (18in) length of waxed string through one of your nostrils and push it out through your mouth. This practice is called neti-kriya. Now I know it sounds like some sort of Japanese torture, but it cleanses the skull and makes the eyes sharp. Since I'm in an environment consisting of manmade light, I have had to fight hard to save my sight from going, hence the wearing of medically prescribed shades. This cleansing action also helps remove diseases above the shoulders. After a bit of practice you should be able to inhale the string with such strength that you can fish the far end out of your mouth. With both ends in your hand you can floss out your nasal passages!

Obviously for me, I can't get hold of string just like that, but I use other things. The more common strings are made from cotton thread, which you dip into beeswax to help stiffen it to allow its entry into the nasal cavity. The beeswax cannot undergo sharp bends without cracking, so I suggest you keep it wrapped or protected to prevent accidental sharp bends getting in the way – it sure makes your eyes water! Even with daily use, I get a month's use out of my string. Hemp strings, if you can get them, are the perfect stiffness and texture but for some of you beginners they may be too eye-wateringly painful! After use they should be rinsed or wiped, and then dried immediately.

Is there a less painful way? For you beginners, I suggest the use of a small rubber catheter. Personally I find this less effective and stimulating, but it is the safest method. Maybe try this first and progress on to the string? With practice, it should be easy to get the string into place. But of course there are gonna be some of you who just can't get away with this cleansing method. Fine, no drama, just leave it out! Before you attempt this exercise, make sure your nose hasn't got anything wrong with it inside. Go see your doctor if you suspect you've got a problem.

How it works – The nasal cavity is like a long cave: it narrows at the roof of the mouth and is widest at the floor.

Keep the string pointed towards the back of the throat, slightly downward and inwards, so that it will smoothly slide through the widest passageway towards the inside back opening of the nose. Don't force it! The idea is that the string will pass through a valve at the root of the nose and into the upper back part of the throat, where it can be grabbed by the index and middle fingers of the opposite hand and then pulled through. Once this has happened, then you can give a gentle massage by pulling back and forth on the string a few times. If pain occurs, then you might be going too fast or maybe the string has become pointed in the wrong direction. Remember, it's not like flossing your teeth! This is a great way of eliminating the disorders of phlegm and produces clairvoyance and clear sight.

Don't throw up! It's important not to insert the fingers too far into the throat to grab the end of the string as this can trigger a reflex gagging action. The end of the string itself touching the back of the throat can also cause this reflex action, so be warned! The entire procedure of inserting the string should only take a few seconds. Have a supply of tissues handy to catch the flow of copious amounts of mucous and always breathe deeply to help yourself relax. In time, your body will react in a less dramatic way when inserting the string.

As an alternative form of neti, try rinsing and cleaning the nasal passages with water – that's the most popular form of neti. It can be used to clear the sinuses or to cure a headache, and it's also said to be good for the eyes. Some people use a small jug with a special spout for this. They stick the spout into their nostrils and let the water run through. It's a good practice if you need it.

At times I just stick my whole face into a bowl of cold water and inhale through the nose and spit the mess out of my mouth. Anyone brave enough to do that first time deserves a medal. Me, I just do it! Although water cleansing or flossing the nasal cavities mechanically removes dust, irritants and impurities from the nasal passages, it has the added benefit of stimulating the nerves, glands and organs of the entire nasal and cranial area, including the eyes, sinuses, ears and cranium. You also can use various healing oils to clean out the nasal passages. Check out what types are available, never use any oil not recommended by a professional. Should you wish to start gently then you should take a mouthful of lukewarm salted water. Bend forwards and relax the soft palate so that the water comes out of the nose.

Air can be an alternative to all this. Exhale completely and then inhale through both nostrils and hold your breath for a few seconds. Blast out the air through both nostrils in short bursts until the lungs are completely empty. Repeat five times. Now close the right nostril using the thumb of the right hand. Inhale, hold for a few seconds and blast out in the same manner. Repeat several times. Next, close the left nostril using the ring finger and the little finger of your right hand. Repeat the above process several times with both nostrils.

HYPERVENTILATION TO GET RID OF CARBON DIOXIDE

Kneel down with the heels together, sit erect and inhale fully. While exhaling in a series of expulsions of the same breath through the mouth (keep your lips puckered as if you are going to whistle), bend forwards and rest your head on the ground in front of your knees. The expulsions are achieved with the help of the abdominal muscles. Come up, slowly inhaling. Repeat several times.

LARGE INTESTINE CLEANSE

Now this one's gonna start cleaning you out from the other end! Usually an enema is carried out with all sorts of paraphernalia, but I'm stuck in a cage so I've had to devise my own method, and it works a treat. I get a dish full of warm water and I squat down so that my rear end is in the water in the dish. I then start contracting and expanding my rectum while churning and drawing the rectum up, which enables my anus to suck up the water into my large intestines. I continue this churning for a while, and then I pump the water out, just like an enema. Of course, you lot will have access to all the equipment. Seek medical advice before having an enema.

There is also an alternative to this method that involves drawing water up into your anus through a bamboo tube, but I draw the line at this. I had a problem allowing a doctor to put his digit up my rear end to check out my prostate gland and prefer to stick my rear end in a dish!

CLEANSE YOUR EYES

Flushing out the eyeballs is important to me coz of what I've already said about my eyes. So how do you do it? Have you ever gazed at something for a long while so your eyes smart and eventually tears fall? Those of you who enjoy freedom can use a candle for this – lucky you! But you shouldn't use a candle that gives off smoke. Ideally, use one of those wick lamps with castor oil because there's no smoke to get in your eyes. Now smoke in the eyes would be annoying. They say crying is a way of releasing certain chemicals that are good for you. Me, I wouldn't know!

LOOK AFTER YOUR COLON
AND FIGHT OFF CANCER

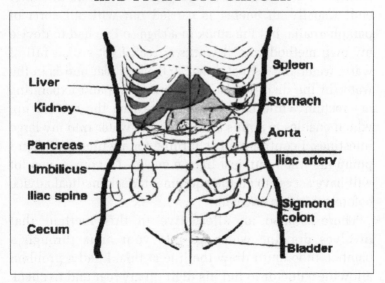

Your intestinal tract begins at your lips and ends at your anus. When the colon is not functioning properly, the entire intestinal tract is affected. Hiatus hernias, peptic ulcers, gastric ulcers, gastritis, stomach cancer, hepatitis, Crohn's disease, gallstones, tumours, haemorrhoids, appendicitis, colitis, gastritis, gastric ulcer, pancreas cancer, diarrhoea and constipation are some of the many diseases directly related to the colon.

Did you know that over 50 per cent of cancer originates from a toxic colon? There is no condition that can disassociate itself from the colon. The healthier the colon, the healthier all other organs of the body will be.

LIFE AND DEATH BEGIN IN THE COLON

The colon is the body's perfect sewage system. A lifetime of eating fast foods and other junk, inactivity, mineral depletion, enzyme deficiency, drinking insufficient water, excessive coffee and alcohol consumption, taking laxatives, overeating and other abuse and neglect makes homeopathic doctors believe that death begins in the colon.

The liver is the main filtration organ of the body and is a powerful organ designed to detoxify any poisons present and remove them from your system. But the problem arises when toxins are present in too great a quantity to adequately be handled by the liver. Phenol, indican and skatol escape the liver's detoxifying action and back up into the lymph and circulatory systems, affecting every organ, gland and system of your body. Most lymph, gall bladder, pancreas and spleen problems can be traced to an inefficient colon.

As with any other organ of the body, when an unusual burden is placed on the liver a breakdown occurs that affects the body as a whole. When the liver is overwhelmed, this type of breakdown results in an increased absorption of toxic substances. Should this condition remain uncorrected, the body slowly begins to poison itself! The lymphatic system is the body's front-line defence against foreign invaders. Like a sponge, it absorbs fluid toxins and potentially harmful bacteria and removes them from the body.

Lymph nodes, like terminal stations, are distributed throughout the body. Most people don't think too much about their lymphatic system until the nodes in their neck, chest, groin and armpits swell up; or the doctor says they've got lymphoma, Hodgkin's disease or some other disease of the lymphatic system. Few orthodox doctors even talk about the relationship between the lymphatic system and the colon. What seems so easily forgotten in our world of wonder drugs, special procedures and cut,

cut, cut, drug, drug, drug society is that both the colon and the lymphatic systems serve as elimination organs. Why do you think the lymph receptor points swell up? It's because your body is full of shit! The lymph nodes are screaming at you, telling you that you're loaded to the hilt with shit! So loaded your body is backed up to the point that it is dumping into receptor sites.

Now where do you think all this garbage is coming from? It's coming from your colon and liver. The lymph is doing its job: it's absorbing toxins like a sponge but even the best sponge in the world can only soak up so much! The fastest way to drain the lymph is to clean your colon by moving the lymph through lymphatic drainage and lymphatic massage. There are herbs to treat the lymphatic system and rebound exercise. A dirty colon will find its way into the lymphatic system. Colonics are the best preventive medicine known for maintaining a healthy lymph system. For you lot who are free, it means you'll all live forever! Me, I just have to wait till I'm free.

Much of your bloating, puffiness, red streaks on the surface of the skin, ankle, leg and arm swelling, sudden weight gain and fluid retention is a toxic condition being neutralised and absorbed by the lymph system. When the bowel is not working efficiently and in a timely fashion, the lymphatic system is forced to work overtime.

COLON HYDROTHERAPY

Colon hydrotherapy is a greatly extended and much more complete type of enema. In water volume alone, one colonic irrigation treatment is equal to 40 or 50 enemas! Whereas a pint to four pints of water is used in an enema, eight, ten, twelve or even fifteen gallons of water is used in a modern-day colonic. Imagine that amount of water blasting out all those toxins, you lucky lot are gonna get all the benefits of this fantastic inner cleansing.

WATER IS THE HEALER

Water is nature's universal cleanser, softener, neutraliser and purifier. Colonic hydrotherapy moves out sluggish faeces, cleans out impacted pockets and begins to soften months and years of hardened plaque. They should make this available on the National Health! Over a period of time water has been known to soften and break stone. Hell, look what it can do to the shoreline! That's exactly how it begins to work inside the walls of the colon. The treatment draws water through the length of the colon and back down again, comfortably and continuously, without the necessity of sitting on a toilet.

Warm water removes strata on strata, layer after layer of hardened faecal material from the walls of the colon, while it dilutes harmful bacteria and toxic concentrations in the large intestine. This cleansing effect reduces stagnation and subsequent bacterial proliferation and also maintains harmony of the intestinal flora while promoting optimal colon health. Rectal/colon cancer is a leading killer. It is the direct result of the typical lazy-arse diet that is high in saturated fat, low in fibre, high in poisons, low in enzymes, high in sugar and low in essential nutrients.

RECTAL/COLON CANCER IS
100 PER CENT PREVENTABLE

In some countries of the world this disease is nonexistent. But some of you have become like overstuffed turkeys and at the same time you're undernourished. In the modern world the average person eats four times the amount they are able to utilise. What's more, their diet is deficient in fibre and essential nutrients. Waste matter that sits in the colon begins to putrefy and rot and over time it begins to eat away at the colon.

Cleansing of the colon minimises exposure of potential carcinogens to the delicate colon tissue. Colon hydrotherapy dilutes the toxin concentration in the colon and facilitates the removal of encrusted waste. The result is a reduced load on the portal (liver) and lymphatic system, allowing the body's elimination channels to open up to their full detoxification potential. When the bowels are blocked, even partially, this slows down the body's entire detoxification process. For a while, other eliminative organs are capable of working overtime but, no matter how strong they may be, the kidneys, lungs, lymph, liver and skin were not designed to do what only the colon can achieve.

LOOK AFTER YOUR COLON AND IT WILL LOOK AFTER YOU

Most skin conditions, kidney disorders, lymphatic congestion, liver sluggishness and blood disorders are the direct result of a toxic colon. Colon hydrotherapy is the direct approach towards correcting most kidney disorders because the kidneys, like the colon, are eliminative organs, meaning they get rid of the crap in your body! Reduce the body's total level of toxicity and you decrease the stress placed on the kidneys.

THE SKIN IS THE BODY'S LARGEST ORGAN

Most skin conditions are directly or indirectly related to the colon. If toxins aren't eliminated in a timely fashion by way of the colon, the body will automatically seek out an alternative channel. Most skin conditions with some fancy medical name attached to them are basically toxins backed up from the colon attempting to eliminate through the skin.

The lungs are connected to the colon. If the colon is not eliminating efficiently, the lungs will attempt to pick up the slack. Most respiratory problems can be traced back to a faulty colon, the root source of most respiratory problems not linked to smoking. Clean the colon and you reduced the body's total level of toxicity, thereby reducing the stress on the lungs, bronchial and respiratory system.

WHAT IS A COLONIC?

You already know what an enema is, or at least you should do. But an enema is very limited in its effect because only a very small amount of water can be introduced into the anal canal and the lower part of the sigmoid colon. It is then necessary to evacuate the bowels after each infusion of water. A colonic, though, uses pure filtered water, which is brought safely, comfortably and hygienically up the full length of your colon and then back down again. Large volumes of water totalling as much as 57 litres (15 gallons) are used over the course of treatment.

In water volume alone, it would take between 40 and 120 enemas to equal one colonic, but the biggest benefit is the therapeutic strengthening effect of every muscle in the colon. The treatment is designed to restore the colon's natural peristalsis, which is often lost after years of faulty diet, constipation or drugs. Indirectly, colonics will help every part of your body. Your colon is your body's sewer system and the health of every cell in your body is related to and dependent on its health.

ENEMAS

The wonderful thing about an enema is that it can be carried out easily and without much preparation. Unless you are severely constipated, an enema should be taken first thing in the morning on an empty stomach and preferably after answering nature's call. There are many types of enema kit available for use in your own home. Obviously I'm not going to recommend a brand!

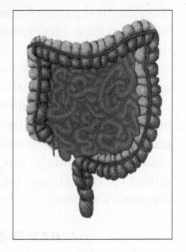

YOUR DIET ON THE DAY
BEFORE ENEMA DAY

Breakfast: Fresh fruit – try papaya, guava, pear, apple, grapes or any other seasonal fruit.
11 am: One glass of seasonal fruit juice.
Lunch: One bowl of vegetable soup, including cabbage, for its high level of potassium.
Evening: One bowl of soup or seasonal fruit juice.
Dinner: One bowl of vegetable soup or seasonal vegetables for roughage.

Note: On that day drink at least 3.6 litres (6 pints) of water. Remember water is one of the four elements and a great healer. Avoid flour and its by-products the day before and on the day you take an enema.

Avoid enemas if you are in any the following categories:
1. Pregnant ladies: in pregnancy (especially up to seven

months), an enema should be strictly avoided as it substantially increases the risk of miscarriage.

2. Persons suffering from extreme piles and or rectal ulcers.

3. Anyone with a history of obstruction in the intestines.

4. Very weak people (after conditions of acute illnesses or otherwise).

THINGS TO AVOID FOR A COMPLETE DETOXIFICATION:

1. Eating bananas the day before and on the day of the enema.

2. Potatoes and similar vegetables

3. Aerated drinks and alcohol the day before and on enema day.

4. Eggs and non-vegetarian food: the day before an enema and on the day.

5. Eating pulses the day before (legumes). You can have them after the enema for lunch that day.
Note: Avoid smoking on enema day and the day before.

So there you have the low-down on how to get a solitary cleanse. My advice to you is to seek out a good private clinic for some colon treatment. All I can manage is a dish of water, so you go for it and enjoy the new you as the old one is flushed out!

SOLITARY DIET

I am probably the world's most natural strongest man and in this *Solitary Fitness* book I've put a workout together that is second to none. Even so, something has been preying on my mind: here I am, stuck in prison, where I have to put up with, and make do with prison food, which I supplement with the few luxuries I can afford to buy. To you, those luxuries are everyday items: honey, fruit juice, oats, raisins and the like. So when it comes to devising a diet plan for you, I'm no expert. It wouldn't be honest or decent of me to pretend I'd written a plan for you when I'm limited in experience of diets for training use.

I admit that I do know probably as much as any nutritionist fresh out of university coz over the years I've built up this knowledge by reading every fitness magazine under the sun. Some were full of shit and others were good mags. I'm not going to personally recommend (or name one), although three mags do stand out from the rest.

For this chapter I've secured the help of guest consultant John Callan. I know a lot of you are going to raise your eyebrows when you find out that he's an ex-power lifter! Why am I using him in my book? I'll tell you why: to give you all the head start you need from an expert. John's not gonna tell you about lifting weights. He'll be telling you the best possible diet for those of you on a low income, who want to eat healthy food. His feature appears further on in this chapter.

Anyway, first let's take diet – *my* diet over my life in prison. I forget what a steak looks like. My diet consists of prison swill, plus stews, curries, spuds, bread, vegetables, fruit and of course porridge. I believe in eating what I can, when I can. It don't matter what you eat – eat a horse if you want – but remember that what you eat you must work off. So think before you eat!

Let's stop all the crap where magazines tell you don't eat that and don't eat this, or that's bad and that's good! You eat what you want! All you need to do is balance it out. Eat as many fruits and vegetables as you can get hold of – and they're cheap, too. I read: 'Don't eat the whole egg: the yolk is full of cholesterol.' Well, I say eat it! Why eat half an egg? What a waste – eat what you like! I don't really want to go on about food and diets coz basically it's commonsense. And I don't want to nag by telling you what or what not to eat, but follow the diet John Callan has worked out for you. His advice is second to none.

Remember this, your body can only keep a low cholesterol count by expelling cholesterol. So, how does it work? Ah, ha, got you there! You see if you drink plenty of water throughout the day then your body sheds excess water it don't need. It's the same with cholesterol. So long as you're active and following my training regime then don't worry about straining off egg yolks – they're too expensive to waste!

PRISON GRUEL HASN'T KILLED ME ... YET!

Just look at my prison diet and ask yourself, has it harmed me? For an average day this is what the prison supply me with:

- Breakfast: porridge, bread and egg.
- Dinner: pie, chips, peas and sponge with custard.
- Tea: stew, bread and fruit.

Over the last ten years, prison diets have got better and we now have a choice. I eat a lot of salads and I drink a gallon of water each day. That's why I sweat and piss a lot, as I'm always cleansing out my body. You're no doubt aware of this after reading the previous chapter. It's why my skin is clear and healthy. I only have one cup of tea a day, though. The tannic acid (tannin) in the tea helps defend my heart from seizing up under pressure.

SOLITARY VITAMINS

OK, you free people, I'm now gonna give you some good tips on vitamins and let you know what's good for you, what food does, etc. Now remember, I'm not a doctor or a dietician. I'm just giving you my knowledge and facts that I've learned in my life and a lot of it is basic knowledge.

VITAMIN TABLETS ARE PISSED AWAY

I read of a major report by Oxford University scientists. It backs up what I've been saying all along. A professor, no less, who headed the research (Professor Rory Collins), said, 'They are safe – we didn't find any hazards, but they are useless.' There you are then! Antioxidants that are claimed to help combat disease are part of the vitamin industry's £175 million income from you lot out there! The report went on to say that you would be better off spending your cash on fruit and vegetables, which contain all the vitamins and minerals you need. Here's a quick rundown on them all:

• **Calcium**: Well, what do you know about it? Calcium is an essential mineral. Who said? I did, and any health book will say the same! Calcium is vital for a good, healthy nervous system. Deficiency can lead to all sorts of problems, i.e. gum disease, muscle cramps, brittle bones, problems you can do without in life. Calcium helps keep bones and teeth strong. Old people are, sadly, prone to calcium deficiency.

So what's best for a good level of calcium? Milk, root vegetables, broccoli, cheese and all other dairy products. Level of dosage? I'm not a doctor but I'll say this: excess dosages will only be excreted away. You can bet it's in multivitamin supplements but, hey, get real. Why take pills or supplements? You're free, get the real thing! Only idiots spend good money on supplements. Get stuck into some good healthy nosh!

Hey, calcium also has its therapeutic uses: it can treat heart problems, insomnia, osteoporosis and growing pains. It can even cure some allergies. Who said? I did! If you don't believe me, go get a health book. Hey, I'm not just a villain, I know these things – I've studied it! Maybe it's not too late for me to become a doctor, but it's the haemorrhoids and other stuff like that I'd get upset with. I can't do that, so it's best that I am what I am. A leopard, they say, never changes its spots! So now let's explain what these vitamins are and what they do.

• **Vitamin B6**: Hey, did you know this is destroyed by

alcohol? It's a fact! But you've got to get real in life: if you took it all too seriously you might as well be a monk! Don't overdo it, life's too short!

• **Vitamin A** – Retinol and Beta Carotene: it's in a lot of animal products, but the beta carotene is the 'plant'. Now take the good old apricot, that's full of it. What does it do? Vitamin A helps you to fight colds and flu. It boosts your immunity. Without it, you'd be in a right state. You'd have bad eyesight, ulcers of the mouth, infections and acne, so get it down your neck coz it can even prevent cancers. Oh yes! Now I don't like liver, but I eat it coz it's full of retinol. Sometimes in life we all gotta eat stuff we don't fancy, especially if you're skint or, like me, in jail! I eat all sorts of crap, but, if it's got any goodness in it, I'll scoff it all and more. I'll shout, 'Give me more of this crap!' Eat plenty of fish, liver, oils, carrots, parsley, spinach and sweet spuds.

• **Vitamin B1** – Thiamine: So what does it do? It's good for the heart and nervous system; it builds muscle and gives you energy. Vitamin B1 actually promotes growth and strength. Get it from porridge, oatmeal, brown rice, vegetables and beans.

• **Vitamin B2** – Riboflavin: Now this is water-soluble (meaning our bodies are unable to store it up, so you need a regular intake) and in times of stress and pressure it's a good source of energy. So what does it do? It's a necessary vitamin for growth and it looks after the skin, hair and nails. Get it down your neck! Oh, I must add that too much coffee or alcohol will destroy this vitamin. Signs of deficiency include a dry mouth, sore lips, insomnia, bloodshot eyes and scaly skin that comes off in flakes. If you're stressed, you should take more of it. Get it from eggs, fish, whole grains and meat.

• **Vitamin B3** – Niacin: Deficiency of vitamin B3 has been linked to depression and even schizophrenia. So what does it do? It fights fatigue and insomnia. Oh, and it also helps convert carbohydrates into energy. It's a fact. It also improves circulation. Get it from avocados (a great source of niacin), lean meats, peanuts, fish, eggs and prunes. Get eating some of these! Oh, and go easy on the prunes. Four or five's plenty. Any more, and that's your problem!

• **Vitamin B–Complex** – Folic Acid: So what does it do? This one is known to be the best for pregnancy as it strengthens the foetus. I read this some years back. You can get it in egg yolks, carrots, melons and fresh oranges.

• **Vitamin B12** – Cobalamin: This is in most foods, so it's not really a big issue unless you're on a vegan diet. If so, you must take supplements. You vegans really amaze me: you defy science! How you can avoid what's natural, I don't know! B12 is good for the red blood cells, but did you know that it also detoxifies? Oh yes, it's awesome! You can find it in beef, kidneys and yoghurt.

• **Vitamin B5** – Pantothenic Acid: I believe this one is the safest of all the vitamins and the good thing is that it produces anti-stress hormones, which are essential for the synthesis of antibodies. You can get it from yeast and green vegetables. Deficiency signs are fatigue, depression, stress and anxiety, bad skin, ulcers and blood disorders. Yeah, all that and more, so get some good vegetables and yeast down your neck!

• **Vitamin B6** – Pyridoxine (Sounds like a poison, eh?): Now I'll put my hands up and say that I know very little on this vitamin, but I do know without it you can get kidney stones. You can find it in bananas, cabbage and eggs. So get some of them down your neck. You don't want kidney stones, do you?

• **Vitamin C** – Ascorbic Acid: This is the main one. Now

remember, it's a water-soluble vitamin and you need a regular intake. You can't overdose on it – your system will piss it out! It helps heal wounds, even burns, decreases blood cholesterol levels, prevents colds and it's even known to stop some cancers. It's essential you get your vitamin C. Find it in fresh raw fruits and vegetables (green peppers, sprouts and cauliflower). If you're bored, make sure you eat a carrot, right?

• **Vitamin E** – Alpha Tocopherol: This is an antioxidant vitamin and it provides the body with oxygen, works as a natural diuretic and improves fertility, among other therapeutic uses. You can get it from wheat germ, soybeans, vegetable oils, whole wheat, oats, almonds, butter and eggs. Signs of deficiency include cataracts, infertility, muscle degeneration and age spots. Not good, eh? Oh, vitamin E skin cream – it's a fact that it slows down the degenerative aging process. Not that I use it. I'm not allowed stuff like that but hell I'd use it if I were free! Why die?

• **Vitamin D** – Calciferol and Ergocaliferol: The body produces this vitamin and you get it through sunlight. Now I must be honest: I don't know how it works, but it does! It's essential for the bones and teeth to develop.

• **Vitamin 'K'** – Phylloquinone or Menaquinone Menadione: Best stick to vitamin K, as you need to be a professor to use such words! Who needs it? Imagine going into a chemist, 'Err, excuse me, could I have some phylloquinone, please?' Sod that! This is a fat-soluble vitamin. You can find it in egg yolks, broccoli, sprouts, leafy greens, green tea, kelp and fish liver oils. Colon disease (not nice to have) and osteoporosis (also not nice) are signs of a deficiency, so get some of that Menaquinone menadione down you!

• **Biotin (vitamin H) Co-enzyme**: Well, I'll tell you now, this vitamin is used to treat hair loss. It's also used in treatment for eczema and it's an organic acid, which contains sulphur. Biotin is essential for fats and proteins to be metabolised by the body. Find it in dairy products, egg yolks, fruit, rice, whole grains, liver and meats.

• **Iron**: This is a mineral nutrient. The iron in your body is stored in your spleen, bone marrow and liver. Amazing, eh? Isn't the body some machine? See why I keep telling you to look after it! You need iron and, without it, you're in trouble. You'll suffer from anaemia, paleness, tiredness, breathlessness – in other words, you'll be worn out! You can get it from red meat, shellfish, liver, molasses, cocoa powder, raw clams and kidneys. Oh, and dark chocolate – plenty of iron in it!

MINERALS AND WHERE TO FIND THEM

• **Magnesium**: Brown rice, chocolate.
• **Zinc**: Offal, meat, seeds.
• **Cobalt**: Milk, clams.
• **Chromium**: Cheese, liver.
• **Copper**: Shellfish, oysters, avocados.
• **Fluorine**: Meat, seafood.
• **Iodine**: Pineapples, raisins, seaweed.
• **Potassium**: Bananas, spuds, soy products.
• **Manganese**: Cereals, bread, nuts.
• **Molybdenum**: Canned beans, eggs.
• **Phosphorous**: Whole grains, soy products.
• **Selenium**: Tuna, onions, broccoli.
• **Vanadium**: Radishes, lobster, lettuce.

MORE GOOD THINGS TO EAT

• **Garlic**: This is the oldest cultivated plant on our planet and used in medicine to prevent coronary disease; it also cleans the blood. Maybe I should have put this one in the Solitary Cleanse chapter? Ah, well, it's here now! Garlic breath? Take raw parsley with it; kills the fumes.

• **Ginseng:** From the East, this root is a source of vitamins, amino acids and trace elements. It helps stimulate the nervous system, lowers blood cholesterol, improves liver detoxification function and improves the appetite. Oh, and it lifts a flagging libido, too!

• **Gingko Biloba:** Chinese, of course. Gotta be, eh? It's the world's oldest tree, been used as medicine for centuries. It contains an antioxidant and is believed to help improve the memory.

I don't want to go too deep into all this as it may confuse you and remember what I've told you: eat sensibly! Really, diet and health is all common sense. I've not mentioned how much of anything to eat, what dosage of vitamins, etc. I'm not a doctor, I don't prescribe anything, I just give you the facts and it's up to you what or how you do it. It's like sex ... I can't show you, can I? You have to do it for yourself!

Get real, face up to life – this is for real! This is the Bronson Solitary Fitness Programme not some Green Goddess shit! Let's go! When you start seeing your health and fitness get better and your bank balance grows, don't forget to send me a card to say thanks, coz I'm after nothing. What you get from Charles Bronson is what you see, I'm a man of honour.

Along with John Callan's support, this is an awesome book that takes you far beyond the boundaries of ordinary fitness and strength training. I will admit that there is only so much I can do on a prison diet of grunge food. Stodgy carbohydrates are no good for building muscle and this is where John lends his expertise. He can confirm and build on what I've already explained. Taking it one step further, the supplements available outside of prison will soon have you as awesome in strength as both John and myself ... well, nearly. I don't want you saying you can't punch holes through bullet-proof glass now!

INTRODUCING JOHN CALLAN

Before you see his record, you need to know a little about John. He's from the Northeast of England and he's one of the most unpretentious men you could ever meet. Try bending steel rods in front of this man and he'll yawn, tearing the *Yellow Pages* in half bores him to tears. What John doesn't know about fitness isn't worth knowing and that's the expertise we're going to draw on for the consultancy side of Solitary Fitness. The pedigree of John Callan is second to none and taking a look at some of his wins is unbelievable stuff:

1988 – Northeast Power-lifting champ, first place in the 75kg (165lb) category.

1989 – Northeast Power-lifting champ, John wins again. He also gets second place in the 82kg (182lb) category of the Yorkshire & Northeast Finals.

1990 – Northeast, and you've guessed it ... first place again.

1991 – First place in the 82.5kg (182lb) category.

1992 – Northeast champ again and also British Bench Press Champion.

1993 – Champ of the Northeast again and first place in the Scottish Open Weight Lifter.

1994 – Third place in the British Championships.

1995 – Northeast champ again. He gets first place in the British Power-lifting Championships and the USA holds the World Championships in Ohio and John gets third place. He finishes off the year by winning the Austrian Grand Prix: first place in the 75kg (165lb) category.

1996 – Mid-England & Northeast champ, first place. The UK Open nets him another first place, now winning the British and European Championships in the same year.

1997 – The European Championships in Germany gets John a first place & Best Lifter award in the 75kg (165lb) category. In the UK Open Championships he wins first place and Best Lifter award.

1998 – European Power-lifting Championships: he wins first place in Germany; wins first place in the European Bench Press and first place in the UK Open. In the World Championships in Graz, Austria, he wins first place (all these were in the 75kg (165lb) class).

1999 – European Championships in France: he wins first place in the 75kg (165lb) class.

YOU ARE WHAT YOU EAT

It is a natural drive of man to want to be strong and well muscled. But if you want to grow muscles you have to feed them with the right stuff. This is what we will talk about here by explaining how the muscles are built, what happens in your body when you train and why you should eat the correct foods and which are those foods.

Muscle tissue contains 70 per cent water, 22 per cent protein and 7 per cent lipids (fats). Therefore, the largest non-water component of skeletal muscle tissue is protein. That is why so many bodybuilders use large amounts of concentrated protein powders and amino acid capsules in an effort to pack on additional muscle mass. As long as you are training with sufficient intensity to stimulate muscle growth, the trained muscles will draw amino acids (the building blocks of proteins) from your bloodstream to increase the mass of the muscles you just stimulated in your workout.

The bloodstream also flushes out fatigue toxins (e.g. lactic acid, carbon dioxide, etc.) and flushes into the muscles new fuel supplies (glycogen, oxygen, etc.). As you see, diet and training are a 50–50 proposition, and only with both together can you achieve the desired results. Muscle gains should be made slowly by consuming plenty of first-class protein while limiting food consumption to no more than 100–200 calories above maintenance level (which for an active 91kg (200lb) male athlete is 4,000 calories per day).

Since your body can digest only 20–25g (¾–1oz) of protein every two to three hours, it makes sense to eat smaller meals more frequently. Rather than two to three heavy meals that an average person consumes, those interested in increasing general muscle should eat five to seven small but nutritionally balanced meals per day. Here is how a small meal nutritional plan should look:

• Morning: protein shake with skimmed milk.
• Mid-morning: low-fat cottage cheese with low-fat yoghurt.
• Lunch: grilled, boned and skinned chicken breast with baked potato and fresh salad (you can add two slices of whole grain bread), one fruit, two cups of water.
• Mid-afternoon: protein shake.
• Dinner: steak (add the juice of half a lemon and sprinkle with black pepper then bake in the oven) with steamed brown rice and steamed vegetables (you can add two slices of whole grain bread), two cups of water or iced tea.

• Late evening: protein shake with skimmed milk.
For at least two of your daily meals, choose a portion of
protein and carbohydrates from each column above plus a
serving of vegetables.

PROTEINS	CARBOHYDRATES	VEGETABLES
Chicken breast	Baked potato	**Broccoli**
Turkey breast	Sweet potato	**Asparagus**
Lean ground turkey	Yam	**Lettuce**
Swordfish	Squash	**Carrots**
Orange roughy	Pumpkin	**Cauliflower**
Haddock	Steamed brown rice	**Green beans**
Salmon	Steamed wild rice	**Green peppers**
Tuna	Pasta	**Mushrooms**
Crab	Oatmeal	**Spinach**
Lobster	Barley	**Tomato**
Shrimp	Beans	**Peas**
Top round steak	Corn	**Brussels sprouts**
Top sirloin steak	Strawberries	**Artichoke**
Lean ground beef	Melon	**Cabbage**
Buffalo	Apple	**Celery**
Lean ham	Orange	**Courgettes**
Egg whites or substitutes	Fat-free yoghurt	**Cucumber**
Low-fat cottage cheese	**Whole wheat bread**	**Onion**

To maintain optimum health, you should consume at
least two servings per day from each of the following five
food groups:

1. Grains, greens, nuts and seeds
2. Vegetables
3. Fruit

4. Milk products and eggs
5. Meat, poultry, fish.

I also recommend a multi-pack of vitamins and minerals (to be taken with a meal) as a means of nutrition insurance against undetectable dietary deficiencies. I advise those who need to lose a bit of fat on their body to achieve that shredded look to cut their calorie intake to 70 per cent of the maintenance level. You could do that by making your protein shakes with water, avoid bread with meals and eat poultry and fish instead of the steak.

Here are some more tips on how to cut a bit more of the fat and the calories in your diet plan:

1. Never fry your foods. You can bake, grill or boil meats.
2. Avoid boiling vegetables (you will lose nutrients). Eat them fresh or lightly steamed where possible without adding butter or oil.
3. Instead of meat, have fish and poultry, which have a low-calorific content.
4. Dry baked potatoes are filling and low in calories. Dry popcorn is also very low in calories and makes a great night-time snack.
5. Avoid full-fat milk and full-fat milk products (cheese, yoghurt).
6. Use a low-calorie dressing for your salads (vinegar, herbs and lemon juice).
7. Avoid sodium in your diet. It retains more than 50 times its weight in water, bloating your body tremendously. Avoid anything with added salt and diet drinks.
8. Avoid spreading butter, jam, etc. on your bread and always prefer whole grain bread.
9. When you get cravings for certain foods not on your

diet, kill them by eating sweet fruits such as
watermelon, sugar melon, oranges and peaches.

If you are wondering which protein supplement to choose
from (there are so many on the market), I personally
would recommend for someone on a higher-budget diet
using Met-Rx (the only product of its type endorsed by
the FDA in USA). One sachet of it (enough for two
servings) contains all the vitamins, minerals and trace
elements you need, as well as a high quality of protein.
For an athlete on a low-budget diet, I recommend you buy
a kilo (2lb) of any whey protein isolate (the Nutrisport
one is quite good and probably the cheapest and most
economical you can find).

For best results I recommend you have your protein
shakes about four times a day:
- First thing in the morning.
- One hour before doing the Solitary Fitness workout so
  as to nourish your muscles before the workout.
- Within an hour of the Solitary Fitness workout. It's very
  important to load your muscles after they have used
  some of the protein taken before and for overall
  recovery.
- And finally just before going to bed. Before, during and
  after training, have a carbohydrate drink to give you
  energy and to supply your body with water as a lot of it
  is flushed out.

Before a heavy workout you could do what is called 'carb
loading' by consuming complex carbohydrates (as a
supplement or as a part of your diet – baked potato, rice) at
least two hours before training. They take longer to break
down in your digestive system and will give you plenty of

slow carbohydrate energy while doing your exercise. If your diet plan allows, 45 to 60 minutes before the workout have a serving or two of simple carbohydrates (chocolate bar), some fruit and a glass of juice. This pre-workout meal gives you the opportunity to blast your muscles for at least two hours without losing any energy momentum.

SUPPLEMENTS ON A LOW BUDGET

As we already outlined the good foods, here we will talk about supplements on a low budget and I will mention the basic supplements your body needs when you are training:

- Proteins – you can find on the market proteins-weight gainers for as little as £10 per kilo (2lb). They will last you about two weeks. This is £5 a week.
- Complex carbohydrate powder should not cost you more than £9 per kilo (2lb). Mix two to three tablespoons of it with about 600ml (1 pint) of water. Add some orange juice for flavour and you will have a quality carb drink ready for when you do your Solitary Fitness workout. It should last you at least four to six weeks, which makes, let's say, £2 a week.
- Multivitamins one-a-day: £1.30 for a month's supply and free-form amino acids as well (about £5 for a month's supply). That is about £1.60 a week.

All together on supplements, let's say, £9 a week.

SUPPLEMENTS ON A HIGH BUDGET

If you can afford them, there are so many products on the market to choose from. Being a professional athlete for many years, I have tried many of them and truly recommend the Met-Rx products. They have been developed by a doctor and are enriched with all the vitamins and minerals your body needs each day. Here is what you will need:

1. Met-Rx protein. It comes in sachets or in a tub. For 20 sachets expect to pay between £30 and £40 (that is about two weeks' supply) and for a tub £23–30 (one month's supply).
2. Met-Rx Mass action – it is a ready powder mixture of carbohydrate, creatine and HMB (good for the arteries) for your own energy drink. Expect to pay £20–28 per tub (enough for one month).
3. Amino acids (as above). And here, £20 should be enough for a week.

But don't go over the top: supplements are a percentage and so is rest and recovery, but intensity of training is very important.

Composed by John Callan, Former World
Power-lifting Champion
Personal Consultations are freely given with each purchase of product by calling John on: 07074 623 623 (UK) or
Contact John by email:
champ1x@hotmail.com

WATER HELPS BURNS OFF FAT

I hope what John has been able to impart to you is of some help. I do appreciate that some of you buying this book will be athletes seeking further guidance. Now, did you know that drinking enough water is the easiest thing you can do to lose excess fat? Best of all, it's free! Don't wait till you're thirsty before having a drink of water. In fact, if you wait until then, your body is already dehydrated because your

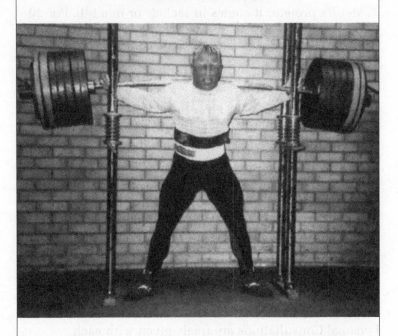

salivary glands are the last resort for getting hydration to your cells. Why do you think the Nomads in the desert suck on a stone if they're getting thirsty when the water supply is running low? Water causes your body to function efficiently.

Fatigue is one of the first signs that you aren't getting enough water. Sometimes you satisfy the need for a burst of energy with coffee, which is the opposite of what you need. Coffee is a diuretic, which actually dehydrates you further, nurturing a self-destructive cycle, and it's the same with alcohol. Drinking sporadically during the day suppresses your appetite. Your hunger for water is the cause of the craving, not the need for extra calories. Thirst signals are often confused with hunger signals. If you aren't used to drinking much water, this could be more of a problem to you than for people who are familiar with the feeling of thirst. People who don't drink water get a small amount from the food they eat, which is not nearly enough. For them, hunger and thirst feels like the same thing, so, along with the tiny bit of water absorbed from food, they also get the unnecessary calories, which are stored as extra fat.

- Water is essential for the body to function properly. It is passed regularly by the body and through the lungs and skin, so it needs to be replaced.
- Thirst is not a good indicator to replace water lost through training or sport.
- The correct way to estimate water losses is to weigh yourself before and after training or sporting activities. The weight lost should be replaced with water.
- During training or prolonged sport, it is best to consume a small glass of cold water at frequent intervals by sipping it.

- In summer the volume of water consumed increases due to losses from increased perspiration.
- A sure sign that you're dehydrated is the colour of your urine. If you're drinking enough water, it should be light yellow to clear in colour. Medium yellowish to nearly orange means you need a drink (any other colour means a trip to the doctor).
- Water helps your liver convert fat into usable energy. If you don't drink enough water, your kidneys are overwhelmed with concentrated fluids and they make your liver do extra work. Your liver works hard to turn your body fat into the energy that you use and, if it has to do the kidneys' work, then you hold on to the extra fat that would have been burned if you'd simply had enough water. And what's worse is that, instead of excreting water and waste products, you reabsorb used water to reuse. This causes water retention and bloating.
- When you don't get enough water, your body panics and holds on to it selfishly as though you're in famine. The best way to get rid of this water retention is to drink enough of it. You'll also feel thirsty more often, and this will start a healthy cycle of thirst leading to hydration. But you have to keep it up because, if you stop drinking enough water, all the good things you've gained from drinking water (balanced body fluids, weight loss, decreased hunger and thirst) will revert back to the way they were.
- Even without changing your eating and exercise habits, increasing the amount of water you drink will cause your fat cells to shrink. Do all three consistently, and you'll easily get to (and maintain) a healthy weight.

> **DON'T PUT OFF TOMORROW WHAT YOU CAN DO TODAY!**

METABOLISM

Let me dispel some misinformation about fitness and fatness. Your body's metabolism is an engine that's always on, whether it's on idle (while you're sleeping) or on red line (when you're working out). If you tune your body properly with training and fuel it properly with nutrition, it's going to be more efficient. Muscle and blood chemistry help each other maintain the metabolic balance through homeostasis, with or without your assistance, but at a price.

People are obsessed with fat, probably because, no matter what some of them try, they're still getting fatter. This obsession doesn't help you get your body to look the way you want it to, and it actually threatens the quality of your life.

YOUR BODY NEEDS FAT TO LOSE FAT

Fact: your body needs fat. Depending on your genetics and metabolic requirements, smart fat should constitute 10–33 per cent of your daily nutritional intake. Fat is actually the symptom, not the illness. A slender, non-fit female on a low- or no-fat, high-carbohydrate diet may be more at risk of difficulties with her metabolism than a slightly overweight, in-shape, middle-aged guy! It's fitness, not fatness that counts. Start paying attention to your shape while you're getting in shape. Stored fat burns last, so measure your inches, not your pounds. Body density is a more important measurement and fitness indicator than body fat because lean muscle weighs more than fatty muscle.

Nerves work in the muscles – they don't work in fat – and it takes four times more energy to move a pound of fat than a pound of muscle.

173

JUMP-START YOUR METABOLISM

No other meal is as important to your overall health and physique as breakfast, although I can't vouch for Sugar Puffs! Your metabolism is on a low simmer while you're snoring the night away. Eating breakfast triggers an immediate increase in calorie burning, which you can sustain all day long. Choose a meal that combines complex carbs with protein, along with some essential nutrients, and you can rev up your metabolism even more and keep your energy soaring for hours. Here are a few metabolic boosters:

- Chromium (peanut butter, cereal, wheat germ): converts blood sugar into energy.
- Vitamin B12 (fortified cereal): helps your body utilise fats and carbs.
- Potassium (bananas, orange juice, peaches, apricots): essential energy producer.

Missing breakfast causes a mid-morning, low-sugar slump, which often results in your grabbing something unhealthy. But high-sugar, high-fat foods only make you moody, fatigued and hungry for more sugar. Show me any kid who doesn't like sugary foods! Sugar is bad in more ways than one, so do your best to limit the amount they eat, especially sweets.

BUILD MUSCLE

The energy you use for your daily tasks and when you exercise is called glycogen and it's stored in your liver and muscles. While you're asleep, your body feeds on liver glycogen, which gets maxed out by morning. Breakfast reverses this deficit. Should you skip the morning meal, your body is instead forced to cannibalise your muscles for energy. Sounds like Bob Maudsley, our very own Hannibal the Cannibal!

ADD MUSCLE, NOT FAT

To build additional muscle, you should eat about 1gm of protein per pound of bodyweight per day, or get approximately 15 to 20 per cent of your total daily calories from protein. The intricate combination is to have enough carbohydrate to spare dietary protein from being used as energy. Availability of all proteins is measured against the protein quality of the egg. The Protein Efficiency Ratio (PER) is measured by the gain in weight of a growing animal over its protein intake. An egg's PER is 1.0. If you eat 7,000 calories, you can get protein wherever you want, but don't have 18 eggs a day.

Complete proteins such as eggs, milk, cheese, red meat, fish and chicken easily supply any athlete's protein requirements, but they may be expensive. Incomplete proteins such as wheat, peanut butter, beans and legumes might take more time to prepare, but it's an effective way to moderate fat intake.

DON'T LET AGE WIN

For those 30+, engaging in Solitary Fitness is the best thing to help you stay as you are. As you get older your body begins to lose muscle mass. Years ago, doctors told you to eat less as you age because 'your metabolism is slowing down'. Middle-aged people do need fewer calories than when they were young adults, but only because the pattern of most people is to lose muscle and replace it with fat as they age, a process that requires fewer calories.

WHAT DOES WHAT?

- Fat – for energy
- Carbohydrate – for energy
- Protein – for growth and repair of tissue

- Water – for regulation of body processes
- Vitamins – for growth and repair of tissue
- Minerals – for regulation of body processes
- Dietary Fibre – for regulation of body processes.

There are two main types of carbohydrates – good and bad

COMPLEX – GOOD	COMPLEX – BAD
Breads, rice, cereals, pasta, potatoes, peas, sweetcorn, parsnip, carrots, dried beans, lentils, fruit, milk & yogurt.	sugar, honey, jams, marmalades, confectionery, cakes, soft drinks, cordials, sweet biscuits, toppings, flavoured mineral water.

EATING DISORDERS

These include anorexia nervosa, bulimia and binge eating. Anorexia nervosa is an excessive concern with being thin, bulimia involves bingeing and then purging what you've eaten (by throwing up, using laxatives, over exercising) and binge eating is overeating that you can't control. I'm no professor, but I can tell you that this sort of thing is a cry for help. It ain't an easy job helping them. So all I will say is they've got my sympathy ... apart from Ian Brady!

BURN OFF 150 CALORIES

- Jumping rope for 15 minutes
- Stairwalking for 15 minutes
- Dancing (fast) for 30 minutes
- Gardening for 30 to 45 minutes
- Raking leaves for 30 minutes
- Swimming laps for 20 minutes
- Walking two miles in 30 minutes
- Bicycling five miles in 30 minutes

- Shovelling snow for 15 minutes
- Bicycling four miles in 15 minutes
- Playing volleyball for 45 minutes
- Touch football for 30 to 45 minutes
- Walking one and three-quarter miles in 35 minutes
- Running one and a half miles in 15 minutes
- Washing and waxing a car for 45 to 60 minutes
- Washing windows or floors for 45 to 60 minutes
- Wheeling self in wheelchair for 30 to 40 minutes.

HOW DOES YOUR BODY MASS MEASURE UP?

Body mass index (BMI) is a measure of the weight a person of a given height can carry and still remain healthy. Here's how you can work out your body mass index:

1. Determine your weight in kilograms. (Divide your weight in pounds by 2.2.)
2. Determine your height in metres. (Multiply your height in inches by 0.025.)
3. Multiply (or square) your height in metres by itself. (For example, if your height is 1.5 metres, multiply 1.5 x 1.5.)
4. Divide your weight in kilograms by the product you got in Step 3.
5. The answer is your body mass index.

Your body mass index should be between 20 and 25. If it is much higher or much lower than that, you might want to hide!

SOLITARY COW PUNCH

Knocking out a cow may seem insane and, to some, impossible. But why is it? A cow's got a jaw and anything with a jaw can be knocked out, if not with a fist then something more substantial. Sure, a cow can't hit back, but what's that got to do with a spur-of-the-moment insane experiment? You, or most of you, eat the things, don't you? No doubt some animal activist is gonna come out of the woodwork and stand with a plaque arguing against this, but it's not really about cows – it's about the power of the punch. It's about hitting the beast on the button, lights out! The cow is just used as an example of how powerful your punch can be. 'His punch was so powerful it would have knocked out a cow' gives the impression that it was indeed one hell of a punch but it didn't mean he went around knocking cows out!

But let me tell you about a punch that can even put a

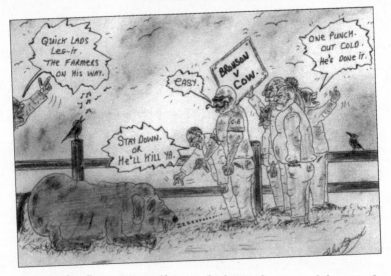

cow on the floor. It's really psychological, a test of the mind and belief. You *must* believe it. If you throw a punch at a cow's jaw then believe it! Have faith in it, or it won't work. Build up, psych yourself up and then let fly with a Cow Punch. I mean, you've heard of a Rabbit Punch? What a weak punch it must be, if it can only be used to knock out a rabbit! Get my drift about the Cow Punch? Mean to knock it out! If you're prepared for it then you'll achieve it. If not, then you'll probably break your fist! It's like smashing through a door, CRASH! When I hit my cow, I hit with 161/2 stone of Cow Thoughts. It's sort of exciting, a test and a challenge. Now I've heard of people on the streets betting each other that they could or couldn't knock out the next stranger out to come along. I frown upon that and the reason for showing you this is purely for defensive use, OK? I actually punched a hole through bullet-proof glass by using this Cow Punch. OK, I damaged the tendons in my arm, but only because my arm got caught on the glass ... my fist was perfectly unharmed!

How do you psych yourself up? Well, I have to go back to the yogi I mentioned earlier, who I met years ago in prison. That man was unbelievable! Anyone seen old episodes of *Kung-Fu* starring David Carradine? Well, this yogi made him look like a new starter! I learned all about visualisation and your inner self, how to cleanse the mind and the body, but I was too unstable to take it all in and use for my own benefit. Hey, I still went through all of the motions, but I just couldn't find the spiritual me ... and then one day, BANG! It hit me for six and I was hooked. I changed my whole ideals, but it was too late. I'd 11 hostages over a period of years while banged up in prison.

For about a year now, I've not been in trouble within the penal system, so, although I've been practising yoga for nearly 20 years, it's only in the last year that I've fully understood what it's all about. I was using it for the wrong reasons, for strength, for pursuing my paranoid thoughts

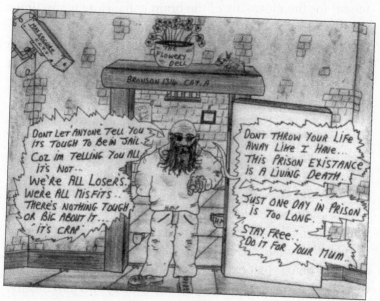

and for every wrong reason you can think of! I've kicked steel cell doors off their hinges, lifted prison governors above my head with the intention of smashing them off the ground and I've ripped so many prison rooftops off that I was given the name 'King of the Roofs'. I've jumped from heights in excess of 30 feet from prison landings just to beat someone up, and some more besides!

Putting all of this to one side for a moment, I can tell you that it just wasn't worth it. I'm going to show you how to find your inner self and make just about anything in your life possible, like the Cow Punch! I was taught a purification exercise called kapalabhati. Although this is given as one of the pranayama exercises, it's good to remember that it is neither a breathing nor a pranayama exercise. What does the word 'kapalabhati' mean? 'Kapala' means 'skull' and 'bhati' means 'to shine'. Although you use your lungs a lot in this particular exercise, it is actually meant for the cleansing of the brain cells. How many times a day, week, month or year that you do this exercise is up to you. It took me nearly 20 years to decide I could use it to my advantage, so it may take you one minute or the rest of your life to feel the benefit in a positive way. Each of us has one thing in common: we're all different to each other. An individual must see if and how often these exercises are necessary. The frequency of the purificatory practice varies greatly. When there is a need, only then do you do these practices. But it is good to know about them.

These practices should be seen as part of the total scheme of self-knowledge. Not only are they supposed to be for the purification of the physical being, but also for the purification of the most vital aspects of the personal, psychological and spiritual being. Just as toxicity is present in the body, then there is also toxicity present psychologically and psychically.

In fact, it is thought that it is ignorance or confusion which has brought about identification with this body, and which in turn has contributed to the physical impurities found in your body. This is the philosophy and psychology behind a technique called nadi-suddhi, which is another method of self-purification. Nadi-suddhi is not strictly a physical exercise but rather a technique of deep psychological and psychic dimensions. It may be regarded as a mystic practice and, as such, it is the inner attitude that is vital to the technique; it should be done with deep feeling and deep visualisation to tremendous effect.

In nadi-suddhi, one visualises a blazing fire that is capable of burning all impurities. Since, in a manner of speaking, the impurities pervade the entire body, and since those impurities must be destroyed without burning up the self or the consciousness hidden behind those impurities, the first step in nadi-suddhi is to visualise withdrawing the jiva (soul).

1. Jiva is visualised at the base of the spine at the muladhara chakra.
2. You then symbolically take the jiva up and visualise it at the very top of the skull. That's only the first stage.
3. When you've done that, visualise whatever defects or weaknesses you may have in you, and visualise them as being concentrated in the spleen region on the left side of the abdomen. You visualise this as some kind of dark force or dark cloud.
4. Then you inhale through the right nostril while you mentally repeat the mantra 'Om'.
5. As the breath is retained, visualise the dark cloud. Exhale through the left nostril.

The recommended ration for inhalation-retention-exhalation is:

- Inhale for 16 (repeating 'Om' 16 times)
- Hold for 64 (repeating 'Om' 64 times)
- Exhale for 32 (repeating 'Om' 32 times).

No doubt a lot of you are going to feel right prats doing this – well, just think of me sitting in my cage doing it! What's really important about this is the visualisation. You see I used to use this to psych myself up before doing something stupid. I'd visualise how I was gonna do it, and it became possible. You must use it to your own advantage.

6. Next, breathe in through the left nostril, mentally repeating the mantra 'yam'. Yam is the 'air' mantra, which is meant to invoke air. You are to entertain the feeling deep within you that, while inhaling and holding the breath this yam is letting loose a gale, which dries up the dark cloud containing those impurities in your body.
7. Hold the breath and feel that the dark cloud has been dried up by the air mantra.
8. Having done this, exhale through the right nostril, repeating the air mantra.

The second stage of nadi-suddhi:
1. As you inhale through the right nostril, the mantra repeated is 'ram', the fire mantra. While mentally repeating the mantra, you visualise that it generates a tremendous fire in the gastric region. It shouldn't be difficult to imagine a fire there. Visualise whatever impurities you may have as being consumed in this fire. It's best to visualise as clearly and realistically as possible. If you want to get rid of anger, for example,

just ask yourself, 'Have I never felt angry or irritable? Of course, I have! All that, I place in the fire.'

2. Whatever you want to overcome is there to visualise. Overcoming fear, overcoming phobias, overcoming low self-esteem. Visualise it, and put it in the fire to be burned.

3. Hold the breath, feeling that all has been burned in the fire.

4. You exhale through the left nostril, repeating the fire mantra. While exhaling, feel as though the ashes from the fire are being blown out.

In the next stage of the cycle:

1. Inhale through the left nostril while repeating the mantra 'tham'. This is pronounced with the same hard 'T' sound as 'tha'. As you mentally repeat 'tham', meditate upon the top of the palate, visualising a lunar orb there, a moon that showers down cool nectar.

2. As you hold the breath and repeat the mantra, you feel that these moon rays of cool nectar shower down to revive your whole system, giving it new shape. The old personality is gone and a new body is taking shape.

3. Exhale through the right nostril repeating the mantra.

You are now ready for the next part:

1. Inhale through the right nostril, mentally repeating the mantra 'vam'. Vam is the bija mantra for water (for the invocation of water).

2. Holding the breath, as you repeat vam, feel that the old, impure body has been destroyed and a new body has been created. Exhale through the left nostril while repeating the mantra. Visualise your new body, see the new you as you wish to be seen.

Now you are ready to move on to the final part of the cycle:

1. Inhale through the left nostril and use the mantra 'lam', which is the bija mantra for the invocation of land (earth).
2. As you hold the breath, visualise a new pure body, solid and ready for the Solitary Fitness routine.
3. Exhale. With your hands in your lap and with the mantra 'soham', visualise the jiva (soul) returning to the muladhara chakra.

That is nadi-suddhi, the mystic practice of the yogis. The orthodox yogis do it before commencing any serious yoga practice. This is what you should be doing before your Solitary Fitness workout, but I don't want to force any of you to do something you don't want to do. It's your decision, but see the benefits you will gain by giving it a try. You can't knock something if you haven't given it a try, can you?

SOLITARY ORGAN

The prospect of increasing penis size is something most men seem to be interested in, if not some women. In fact, according to varying sources I've studied, it would seem that anywhere between 90 and 95 per cent of you aren't happy with what you have. But did you know that 90 per cent of men, regardless of race, possess roughly the same erect penis length of around 15cm (6in)?

Penis size is usually the butt of shower jokes, maybe that's why some men just don't do sports ... it's not doing the sports, it's the showering afterwards in a multi-use changing room that puts some men off. This can damage a man's self-esteem, his confidence and his perception of his masculinity. They say women are less concerned, and rank penis size fairly low on the list of important physical attributes in a man. Of course, these reports would say that, as men probably write them! Durex, the condom manufacturers, carried out a survey and found that 60 per cent of women are unhappy with the size of their partner's penis. Whether this is the case or not, penis size is definitely more of an issue for men than women.

So here I am, in my nice warm cage, talking about things I can only dream of. I wonder how many of those sex therapists out there really care about such matters? Well, I care what happens to my students of Solitary Fitness and every part of your body counts. My findings are that there is no fast wonder cure to enlarge the penis. Surgery is dangerous and vacuum pumps only engorge the penis with blood for a limited period of a few hours, giving the illusion of a larger penis when flaccid. When erect, it is no larger than previously.

PENIS FACTS

- The average penis size when erect is only 15cm (6in) and 90 per cent of men possess this size.
- In the UK it is estimated that millions of men suffer from impotence (erectile dysfunction).
- Having weak erections is the first sign of urinary and prostate disease.
- Most men can't have intercourse for longer than five minutes before ejaculating due to a weak, underdeveloped PC (pubococcygeus) muscle.
- Most men have very poor blood circulation to the penis and testicles.
- By the age of 27, 95 per cent of men cannot have one-fifth of the erections they had when they were 20.
- 85 per cent of women NEVER achieve an orgasm during intercourse and 72 per cent said they have lied to their lover about having an orgasm.

- 100 per cent of men have a weaker, smaller, underdeveloped penis compared to what they could possess.
- By the age of 50, eight out of ten men have cancer cells developing in their prostates.
- A larger penis has much more surface area and is capable of stimulating more nerve endings, providing more pleasure for you and your partner.
- A man endowed with a 18 or 20cm (7 or 8in) penis is simply better equipped than a man with a 12 or 15cm (5 or 6in) penis.

PENIS PUMPS

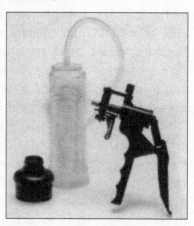

These work by creating a vacuum around the penis. They consist of an acrylic cylinder, into which the erect penis is placed. At the base of the cylinder an airtight seal ensures the vacuum created is maintained. Through the use of either an electric or hand pump, the air within the cylinder is then extracted and the resulting vacuum forces increased volumes of blood to be drawn into the penis. This increased volume of blood in turn causes the erect penis to temporarily swell in size.

DON'T WASTE YOUR MONEY!

The results achieved in erection size are often similar to those experienced during extreme sexual arousal, when the penis is engorged with blood to its full capacity. Although pumps certainly engorge the penis to capacity and result in immediate gains, the effects as mentioned above are in the main only temporary and are lost within a few hours. Unfortunately for you, the use of a penis pump does not result in sustained long-term improvements in penile size. Penis pumps have no effect in increasing the natural capacity of the erectile chambers, which is a necessity, if permanent gains are to be achieved.

THE DANGERS OF USING PUMPS

There are no well-documented scientific studies of the long-term effects of pumping. However, excessive pumping or the use of a too-intense vacuum can have detrimental side effects. Lymph blisters are common and men often notice a reduction in sensitivity and problems achieving firm erections. Moreover, burst or ruptured blood vessels can lead to bruising and at worst haemorrhaging. So take my advice, leave them out of your Christmas list!

Having a small penis makes you feel inferior and embarrassed. Confidence with women and sex will be low. It has been proven time and again that sexiness comes from confidence. Having a bigger, thicker and more muscular penis will give you that confidence. Learn how you can develop your penis so that in future years you are still having an active sex life.

THE BENEFITS OF PENIS EXERCISING

1. Better sex.
2. It cures impotence.
3. Longer-lasting sex.
4. Improved circulation.
5. Superior control over ejaculation.

6. Increased semen and ejaculation flow.

7. Increased sex drive and stamina.

8 Straightening of a curved penis (Peyronies disease).

PENIS ENLARGEMENT EXERCISES

Although I've no use for a larger penis, I can only guess from the survey results that most of you guys reading this will want a bigger tool. Which reminds me of a joke ... This guy comes across a magic lamp; he rubs it and out pops the genie of the lamp. The genie grants the man only one wish. The man says, 'I wish my dick trailed along the ground.' The genie granted the man's wish ... the man's legs fell off!

There are a number of ways you can produce penile enlargement via exercise, but not like the geezer below!

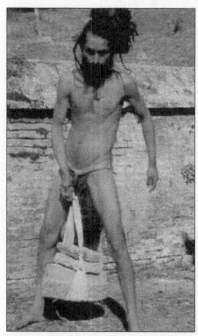

Not a recommended exercise for penis development!

Penis exercises work on the basis of exercising the muscle structures of the penis, known as corpus cavernosumwhich makes up two-thirds of the penis. Your current penis size is determined by the maximum amount of blood that your corpus cavernosa can hold when you have an erection. With proper exercise, the corpus cavernosa can be developed to be larger and stronger so that it will be able to hold more blood, giving you an increase in penis size. The corpora cavernosa is a spongy tissue containing distensible blood spaces, which increases in size when blood is pumped into it. It is similar in construction to the pore cells in marine life called sponges. When the pore cells in a live sponge are repeatedly stretched, its absorption pores expand and heal in this expanded state. Thus, the pore cells become larger and more capable of absorbing more water and nutrients.

THE THEORY ON HOW TO OBTAIN A LARGER AND STRONGER PENIS

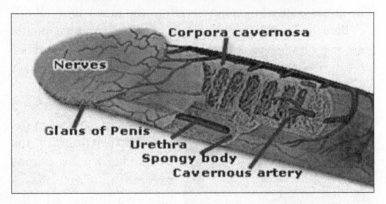

As I've said, the corpora cavernosa is a live tissue that responds similarly to a sponge. Therefore, the actual size of the erectile tissue increases as the distensible blood spaces increase their ability to absorb more blood under the continuous stretching and healing of exercises. Thus, a larger penis can be achieved via exercises.

Recent studies conducted by scientist D J Millward have shown that muscle cells, including the corpora cells within the penis, are snugly surrounded by thin sheaths of connective tissue considered to be similar to tough layers of plastic wrap.

CONNECTIVE TISSUE MUST BE STRETCHED

For each cell to enlarge, these connective tissues must be stretched. Your body responds to physical stimulation and exercises by growing and adapting to changes and the various stressors exerted. Due to this innate ability, muscle fibres stretch and grow to accommodate exercise, along with the tendons and ligaments. The penis is not made up of muscle tissue, but the ligaments attaching it to the pubic bone affect it.

HOW TO INCREASE THE SIZE

To increase the size and especially the length of your penis, the connective layers that surround the erectile tissue have to be stretched. This is where penis exercises come into place, helping you to stretch the connective tissues surrounding the erectile tissue. These pre-existing cells in your penis are forced to increase a small amount in size each time the exercises are performed, giving you a larger and more muscular penis over a period of time.

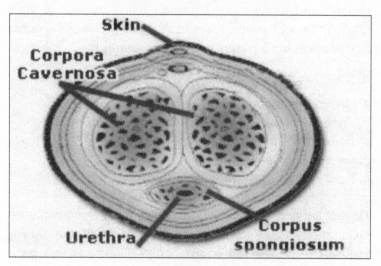

The corpus cavernosum is a certain size and so limits your erection length and width. The exercises described in this section force blood to fill all spaces within it, stretching and enlarging the blood spaces with every session. This stretching tears down the corpora cavernosa, causing it to grow back much larger and stronger than before.

MY CAVEAT

These exercises are not intended to treat medical conditions. As I've previously said, I'm not a doctor, so, if you experience any pain or discomfort during the routine, stop immediately and consult with your doctor. Neither my publisher John Blake Publishing nor I is to be deemed liable for any injuries or health problems encountered directly or indirectly as a result of these exercises. It's important to address any concerns you might have about these exercises to your doctor before you start. But I can advise that I do all of the exercises listed within this chapter and many more I haven't listed for fear of your copying them. I mean, I wouldn't want you to get a penis that was too big for your pants now, would I?

BASIC CONDITIONING EXERCISE

1. Get your manhood erect.
2. Put a towel or T-shirt over it and hold it up in mid-air. If you can't do this then you're a pussy!
3. Let your pulse move it up and down.
4. Now start to lift it up with willpower. Up ... down!

Do this for as many reps as you can. It also cures premature ejaculation. How? Simple: control! Imagine the power within (it can only make sex better). Good sex is a great workout, making you sweat and burning off calories. But I'll settle for the towel technique. I'm not greedy, see, or a stud, but the women I've had will confirm that a good, hard tool works better! That's it, lads – good lifting!

GIRLS! If you read this, which you probably did, don't get your fellas lifting nothing too heavy. Why? Believe it or not, the veins can get damaged. So don't be pushing your man too hard coz it may cost you in the long run. The penis is no different to a bicep, so treat it kindly. In fact, when your man has completed the towel technique, why not give it a good massage, plenty of oils and give it the once over? We all need a bit of praise, or a pat on the back at times – all that lifting is bloody hard work!

MAIN CONDITIONING EXERCISES –
JELQ TECHNIQUE

Before you start your workout, make sure you apply a warm towel to your penis to prevent bruising. Soak a towel in warm water, bring your penis to an erect state and gently wrap the towel around it. Leave for approximately two to three minutes. Now follow the exercises below every other day.

1. Without causing pain, firmly grip your penis just below the head. Pull it out directly in front of you until you feel a stretch at the base and the middle.
2. Once your penis is stretched to a comfortable distance, hold it there for approximately 12 to 15 seconds.
3. Repeat Steps One and Two for 15 repetitions.
4. Once you are finished with the steps, swing your penis in a circular motion for approximately 20 seconds.
5. Now bring your penis to a semi-erect state.
6. Apply lubricant oil on both hands and on your penis.

7. Without causing pain or discomfort and with your thumb placed directly on your forefinger, firmly grip around the base of your penis.
8. Keeping a firm grip, slowly slide down the length of your penis until you reach the middle.
9. Repeat the cycle, alternating hands. Perform 100 slides with each hand. Each sliding (milking) motion should last approximately three seconds.

Penis enlargement remedies have been around for thousands of years. Ancient sexual manuscripts such as the Kama Sutra have various concoctions and exercises for enlarging the male sex organ, but the results offered by modern medicine appear more reasonable. Exercises to stretch the penis are another common component of a well-planned routine. They work on the well-known principle of the body being capable of adapting when subjected to the force of tension. In fact, the application of tensile force is used in certain areas of mainstream medicine and is actually part of the post-operative treatment for men who have undergone penile augmentation surgery (phaloplasty). These techniques primarily stretch the suspensory ligaments responsible for supporting and connecting the penis to the pubic bone. The suspensory ligaments also secure approximately half the length of the penile shaft within the body. Stretching these ligaments encourages the part of the penis usually held within the body to be gradually exposed over a period of time.

Interestingly, surgical techniques to lengthen the penis also focus on the suspensory ligaments. However, instead of stretching the ligaments, they are literally severed. This results in immediate gains in length but it is a far more drastic procedure. One of the main drawbacks of surgical lengthening procedures is that the formation of scar tissue can actually cause the suspensory ligaments to heal so they are shorter than they were originally and initial gains can be partially or totally lost.

Stretching exercises are usually performed when the penis is flaccid. The basic technique involves gripping the penis firmly around the head and then gently pulling forward. The idea of the stretch is not to pull the penis to the point of pain but sufficiently so that it is stretched to its maximum comfortable limit. An example of a stretching exercise would then be to hold the stretch for approximately 15 seconds before relaxing. To complete the session the process would then be repeated ten to fifteen times. One thing to bear in mind is that stretching exercises only promote gains in penis length and will not increase penis girth. These techniques only form part of an effective routine.

DON'T BE FOOLED BY PENIS ENLARGEMENT PILLS!
Ingredients will vary, depending on the company you purchase from. Some of the more commonly found herbal components of enlargement pills include ginkgo biloba, saw palmetto, epimedium sagittum, catuaba, cuscuta seed, horny goat weed, maca root, yohimbe and muira pauma. All the stuff you can get off the shelf! In fact, beware of some of the contents as they can cause you harm. Don't be a pill merchant!

HYPNOSIS
Time to let the editor of this book have his say. Steve Richards is also a qualified clinical hypnotherapist. He tells me there are inner blocks or beliefs that may have contributed to stop your penis from growing! Penis

Enlargement Hypnosis, as in Breast Enlargement Hypnosis, will clear away all those inner blocks so that you can actually enlarge your penis size permanently. Of course, this doesn't work on organs that have become stunted by virtue of some sort of trauma.

As much as impotency and premature ejaculation can be treated by hypnosis, so can an underdeveloped penis. Prior to working on the problem, the subject is taken into a deep trance and the subconscious mind asked if it is safe to proceed and if it is the right time to tackle the problem. Depending on the answers, treatment can start or may be suspended. It's just like losing weight – some people just can't seem to lose weight or will gain back whatever they lose in a matter of months. This is due to the fact that the mind had been programmed to accept the fat you and not the skinny one. At first it may sound odd to think that hypnosis could change your body size or shape, or enlarge your penis, but it is true. This has already been proven by thousands of men around the world. There is plenty of scientific evidence about the existence of mind–body connection and how we have our own 'inner physician' who can dictate the growth and dismissal of specific cells within our body. As much as hypnotic death can shut down your body, so it can also be brought back to life by hypnosis.

PUBOCOCCYGEUS – LOVE MUSCLE

Both men and women have a PC (pubococcygeus) muscle and it is responsible for the health of the pelvic floor. Trust me, that's not all it's used for. You have to keep this muscle in tip-top shape to maximise your sexual experiences. The next time you go to the toilet and begin urinating, try to stop the flow midway. Can you? If not, then you need to start exercising as soon as possible to maintain penile fitness. Another test is when you have an erection. Can you make your penis jump substantially? Exercising this muscle regularly prolongs the duration of lovemaking and will make your climax much more intense. Remember the towel-raising exercise mentioned earlier? Healthy PC muscles can actually allow you to raise and lower the towel at will.

The PC muscle surrounds the penis, prostate and anus. It runs from the pubic bone to the tailbone in a figure of eight around the genitals. Because it helps to control many aspects of sexuality, it is also known as the 'love muscle'. It plays a vital role in sexual response – the jolts and spasms of orgasm are actually caused by involuntary contractions of the PC muscle. The exercises used to strengthen the PC muscle are known as Kegels. They were initially intended to benefit women with poor bladder control, but their effect on improving the sexual health of men has become widely accepted. Kegel, or pelvic floor, muscle exercises help strengthen weak muscles around the bladder. When these muscles are weak, urine can leak from the bladder.

PELVIC FLOOR

The pelvic floor is a hammock of muscles that supports the internal abdominal and pelvic organs. These muscles run in different directions and are of different sizes. Their job is to support, lift and control the muscles that close the urethra (the tube that urine passes through). You exercise these muscles by squeezing and relaxing them. This takes effort and practice!

ISOLATE THE PC MUSCLE!

To make sure that you are exercising the right muscles, try starting and stopping your urine stream. This exercise will help you find the correct muscles. Repeat once a week to check whether or not you are using the right muscles. Do not tighten your buttock or thigh muscles when doing these exercises. Relax your stomach muscles as much as possible.

> **TIP**
> When standing, squeeze your pelvic floor muscles and you should see your penis move slightly.

THE MALE PC MUSCLE

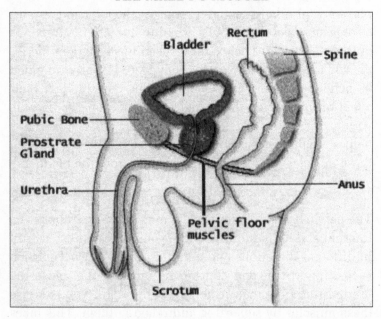

The PC muscle is the key to more powerful, pleasurable and forceful orgasms, stamina in lovemaking and ejaculation. It helps hold the contraction for longer and you experience more powerful contractions. This muscle also helps you retain your erection after ejaculation, develop a richer blood supply to the penis and nerves, and increase your sensation. Make your penis jump when thrusting into your partner – a pleasant experience for both! Exercising the PC muscle means improved prostate health and it also improves the way you perform sexually. Squeezing well-toned PC muscles helps to bring women to orgasm during sex; no more premature ejaculations, firmer erections. It helps to cure impotency, too.

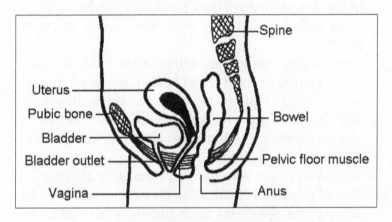

THE FEMALE PC MUSCLE

Pelvic floor muscles can become weak and sag because of childbirth, lack of exercise, the change of life or just getting older. Weak muscles give you less control and you may leak urine, especially with exercise or when you cough, sneeze or laugh. The muscles of the pelvic floor are kept firm and slightly tense to stop leakage of urine from the bladder or faeces from the bowel. When you pass water or have a bowel motion, the pelvic floor muscles relax. Afterwards, they tighten again to restore control. Loss of muscle tone can lead to incontinence, so get working on it now, coz I do!

HOW TO LOCATE THE PC MUSCLE

1. Sit comfortably with your knees slightly apart. Now imagine that you are trying to stop yourself from farting. To do this, you know that you have to squeeze the muscle around the back passage. Try squeezing and lifting that muscle as if you really do have wind. You should be able to feel the muscle move. Your buttocks and legs should not move at all. You should be aware of the skin around the back passage tightening and being pulled up and away from your chair. Really try to feel this.

2. Now imagine that you are sitting on the toilet passing urine. Picture yourself trying to stop the stream, really try to stop it! Try doing it now as you are reading this. You should be using the same group of muscles that you used before, but don't be surprised if you find this harder than the previous exercise.

3. When you empty your bladder, voluntarily stop the flow of urine mid-stream. The PC muscle contracts to achieve this. Now relax again and allow the bladder to empty completely. You may only be able to slow down the stream. Don't worry, your muscles will improve and strengthen with time and exercise.

TIP

If the stream of urine speeds up when you try to do this exercise, you are squeezing the wrong muscles! Do not get into the habit of doing the stop test every time you pass urine. This exercise should only be done once a day at the most. Now you know what it feels like to exercise the pelvic floor!

Now you've located the PC muscle do these!

1. Tense your PC muscle and hold the contraction for two

seconds before relaxing. Do 20 reps, three times a day.

2. Tense your PC muscle slowly and hold the contraction for five seconds before relaxing slowly. Do ten reps, three times a day.

3. Tense your PC muscle and hold the contraction for ten seconds before relaxing. Do ten reps, three times a day.

4. Tense your PC muscle and hold the contraction for 15 seconds before relaxing. Do ten reps, three times a day.

ROUTINE

1ST WEEK	NO. 1 ONLY
2nd and 3rd week	No. 1, followed by No. 2
4th and 5th week	No. 1, followed by No. 3
6th week onwards	No. 1, followed by No. 4

Continue doing the PC muscle exercises to strengthen and keep the muscle in optimal condition.

MORE PC EXERCISES

There are different sets of exercises you can do. Select the one that suits you and do it regularly. Tell your woman to do the exercises, too – they will have the same beneficial results. Always keep in mind that you should keep your other muscles relaxed.

EXERCISE ONE

1. Quickly clench and unclench your PC muscle for ten seconds. Take a break for ten seconds. Perform three sets and then take a 30-second break.

2. Clench and unclench for five seconds with five-second breaks in between, ten times in a row.

3. Tighten your PC muscle for 30 seconds and release for 30 seconds, three times in a row.
4. Repeat the first step and you're done for the day!

EXERCISE TWO

1. Tighten your muscle and hold for a count of five and then release. Repeat ten times.
2. Squeeze the muscle fast ten times. Repeat three times.
3. Tighten and release your PC muscle in long and short intervals for counts of ten. Repeat three times.
4. Squeeze your muscle and hold it for as long as you can. Try to work your way up to 120 seconds. Relax, that's only two minutes!

EXERCISE THREE

1. Squeeze and release your muscle over and over again. Begin with a set of 30, and then slowly work your way up to over 100.
2. Squeeze as deeply as you possibly can. Hold it for 20 seconds and then rest for 30 seconds. Repeat five times.

EXERCISE FOUR

Simply begin squeezing and releasing your muscle for two minutes a day and gradually work your way up to doing this for 20 minutes at least three times a day. You should eventually be able to perform at least 200 repetitions per session.

TIPS

- Get into the habit of doing your exercises in conjunction with other things you do regularly. If you're a housewife, try doing them each time you put your hands in water; if you're at the office, every time you answer the phone, whatever you do often. Do the stop test once a day when passing urine. This should get faster and easier.

- Ladies, if you are unsure that you are exercising the right muscle, put one or two fingers in the vagina and now try the exercises to check. You should feel a gentle squeeze if you are exercising the pelvic floor.

- Use the pelvic floor when you are afraid you might leak: pull up the muscles before you sneeze or lift something heavy. Your control will gradually improve.

- Drink normally, at least six to eight cups of water every day. I drink a gallon of the stuff every day! And don't get into the habit of going to the toilet just in case. Only go when you feel your bladder is full.

- Watch your weight – excess weight puts extra strain on your pelvic floor muscles.

- When you have regained control of your bladder, don't forget your pelvic floor. Continue to do your pelvic floor exercises a few times each day to ensure that the problem does not come back.

- A scientific study was done to find out the best way for men and women to completely empty their bladders. They discovered this was to sit on the toilet – even us men – lean forward and put your hands on your knees and then start to urinate, holding until empty.

- It usually takes six to twelve weeks to see exercise gains.

- Practise squeezing these muscles when you're watching TV, queuing or driving your car.

- Some people exercise more than they should, hoping they will regain bladder control more quickly. If you exercise too much or too soon, your bladder control may get worse for a while. Start slowly and increase the amount of exercise slowly.

You can do pelvic floor exercises wherever you are – no one need know what you're doing!

PC EXERCISES FOR MEN

Always squeeze your pelvic floor muscles when you sit up from lying down, stand up from a sitting position, or lift something heavy.

SOLITARY FAT LOSS

Did you know there's a guy in the USA who tried to sue fast-food restaurants for making him fat? Sadly, Caesar Barber blamed McDonald's, BurgerKing, Wendy's and Kentucky Fried Chicken for contributing to his obesity, claiming that, because these restaurants advertised their burgers as '100 per cent beef', he thought they were healthy. What's worse is that there are plenty of fat people who, like him, want to spread the blame for their weight problems, from being stretched for time to being too ill to exercise! Get real, fatties are just too lazy to exercise! Before you start playing the blame game, work out what's standing in the way of your weight loss.

I'm going to say exactly what I said to you in the Solitary Commitment chapter fat people actually smell and they fart a lot! They're unhealthy and they're sluggish. Look, I'm not gonna mess with you, fat people

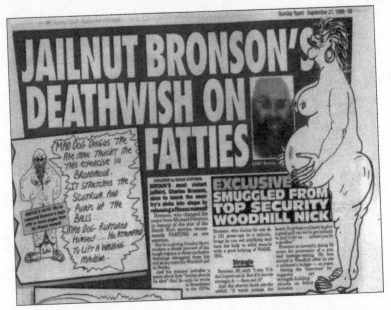

have got to want to change. If you're one of them, then start making that change right now, not tomorrow! Go to your food cupboard and fridge. Be brave, throw all you know is useless into the bin, or give it to a poor neighbour who ain't got the likes of what you're about to chuck out. You've probably got enough fat on your body to keep you alive for a month. If you're fat, then it's a fact, I'm not gonna pretend! You're sluggish, you're lazy and you're a joke! End of quote.

WHY YOU ARE FAT

Obesity is on the rise, despite the media's obsession with six-pack abs and movie-star bodies. There are many things that contribute to your current weight problems including:

1. Cars.
2. Busy schedules.
3. Computers and the Internet.

4. Hours of mindless TV-watching.
5. City councils that aren't exercise-friendly.
6. Technology that makes it possible to do everything from a chair.
7. Exercise is scary. You might do it wrong, you might fail, you might hurt!
8. Medical advances that let you off the hook such as plastic surgery or liposuction.
9. Lack of physical activity in schools as well as easy access to junk food for your kids.
10. You believe that, if you can't meet the standard exercise guidelines, why exercise at all?
11. Denial. Most people know that quick-fix pills and gadgets don't work, but they keep trying them anyway to avoid exercise.
12. Confusion. There are so many rules about eating and exercise that you allow yourself to get overwhelmed by the choices and don't do anything.
13 Fear of being liked so you remain fat (ugly)!

WEIGHT-LOSS SUPPLEMENTS ARE TOTALLY WORTHLESS!

I'm gonna show you how to blast that fat off without the use of supplements or drugs or equipment. For years you've had it pounded at you that there is a wonder drug that will burn all your fat away, but I say all ineffective pills, powders and equipment are a needless waste of your good money! Spend all you want on these magic pills, sure they might burn a few calories off you, but it will not be permanent fat loss ... it will return, twice as ugly!

Stop wasting your time on these rip-offs and gimmicks – they're never gonna work! There are no miracle results. You just ain't gonna burn that ugly fat arse off, or those bun hips. You've probably bought a whole load of these gimmicks over time and maybe you've got an ab machine in the back of your wardrobe. Take it out now and throw it away! They're worthless, probably an antique in time.

OK, you're confused; I can take that! You've been led down the garden path by a bunch of cowboys and you believed them. Body fat knows no bounds. It will attach itself to every part of your body like a barnacle clings to the underside of a boat! Look, I was once just as chubby ... yeah, I was up to 20 stone in weight!

WEIGHT-LOSS LIES

Listen, what I want to know is how these companies can get away with telling you lies. I read about their outrageous claims with my own eyes. Unproven claims are thrown at you. OK, there are strict advertising laws but there's always one that sneaks past them and has your hard-earned cash taken from you in a flash, and that applies worldwide. I get newspapers and magazines from across the globe sent to me by my friends and I'm amazed people can get away with the claims they make. Supplement providers rarely have challenges made to their outlandish claims. You accept what they say, and you're all sheep! They make claims that you can look like Arnie in a few weeks or promise to show you how to develop rock-hard abs in one month or shed a stone of ugly fat in one week. It's all lies!

Look, if these products actually worked, do you think the companies would remain in business? Think about it! There would be no more fatties in the world to sell their products to. But no, they prey on your weaknesses and want you to stay fat so they can keep selling their lies to you, and you keep on buying them!

EAT LESS AND GET FATTER

Starvation diets are a waste of time. All that happens is that your body starts to cannibalise itself and eats valuable muscle mass instead. Yes, you get slimmer but a lot of the initial weight loss is water and muscle. The aim of the game is to burn off ugly fat, not pretty muscle. When you punish your body by withholding calories from it for as little as several hours, your body goes in to starvation mode, which reduces the rate at which you burn fat. On such routines you'll not only suffer from very low energy levels but also your body-fat percentage will actually increase when you return to a reasonable food intake. Sounds familiar? This is called yo-yo dieting. It comes off, and it goes back on! Your weight will drop, but muscle and water will comprise a large percentage of the weight loss and reverting to normal quantities of food yields rapid body-fat increase. Don't ever forget this! Diet routines focusing on calorie restrictions or starvation are actually bad for you!

FAT PEOPLE USUALLY EAT LESS THAN NORMAL-SIZED PEOPLE

Have you ever noticed how most fat people actually consume very few calories relative to their size? They may eat two or three small meals per day, yet actually end up putting on weight over time. Why? Reduced calories! Yes, if you eat properly, you can actually consume more food while still losing weight.

Of course, you shouldn't overeat or stuff yourself with junk. Start by eating sufficient food to feel satisfied. Severely restrictive food plans automatically prompt the body to slow the rate at which it burns energy, which literally dissolves all chance of body-fat reduction. Eating more while losing weight? Yes, it really does work! Sharply reducing calories is not the answer to losing unwanted body fat. In fact, it will actually cause your body to manufacture fat-storing hormones!

PLAN YOUR MEALS

When you're away from home and you feel your stomach rumbling, chances are the most readily available options will be of the junk-food variety. Chances are you will succumb to the burger and chips scenario unless you plan ahead. But to lose weight, you have to start to anticipate hunger pangs and carry convenient, nutritious snacks such as dried fruit and whole-grain cereal bars. Plenty of fruit is good and cheap, and it fills you up.

INCLUDE FAT IN YOUR DIET

Ironically, the very thing you want to burn off can help you burn it off, and that's FAT. Always include a little fat, which is the slowest digesting macronutrient of all. Add an ounce or two of grated cheese, etc., and your gut will shush till dinner. Or try a tablespoon of reduced-fat peanut butter on celery stalks. None of these munchies will cost you more than 250 calories and 6g of fat.

NOTHING IN POWDER OR PILL FORM CAN HELP

Companies continually advertise amazing results yet deliver nothing but the status quo. OK, drink a low-calorie meal replacement drink for the rest of your life! Once you start down that path, then that's the path you'll stay on!

EXERCISE ALONE WILL NOT LOSE FAT

The only real required element for consistent fat loss is proper diet, thus exercise is not an essential factor. How can I say that? Look, I'm here to help, not to hinder you! All I will say is that if you want to accelerate fat loss then exercise along with proper food control can do this. For example, if you lose 15 pounds in one month through proper diet techniques and no exercise, you will enhance results by five to 15 pounds (losing 20 to 30 pounds) through introducing proper exercise variables in conjunction with diet. Thus, if you wish to enhance the rate of progress, adding exercise to proper diet is a worthwhile technique. Yet exercise is not necessary.

WEIGHT-LOSS CENTRES

I don't have any specific arguments with weight-loss clinics, but I firmly believe that anyone can lose weight without their symbolic handholding techniques. OK, you want some support to see you through? Put a mirror in every room of your flat/house/caravan or wherever you live. That will be your friend! These fat-loss clinics charge a mint for being a coach while you are putting in maximum effort – they should be paying you for working your fat off!

THE WRONG WAY TO HIT A BRICK WALL

A low-carbohydrate diet plan will cause a reduction in body weight (five to ten pounds) within the first one to two weeks, but the majority of weight lost is, as I've already said, muscle, and water, not fat! This is followed by no further weight loss. The initial reduction of water/muscle actually slows down your metabolism (the rate at which you burn calories) so you find that body-fat levels stay constant and you hit a brick wall!

A SMALLER YOU ISN'T A MORE BEAUTIFUL YOU

Losing muscle tissue and water weight won't tone your muscles up, nor does it improve your appearance. In fact, it greatly slows or even prohibits the fat-loss process! In addition, weight loss on a low-carbohydrate plan produces a smaller version of your former self rather than enhancing your physical appearance due to muscle loss, which eliminates tone and creates a sagging, unappealing body structure. On a low-carb diet plan, every lost pound returns! So leave well alone! No doubt some of you have already been down this road ... it's a slippery one at that!

MUSCLE, WATER AND FAT

Body weight is composed of water, muscle and FAT! Your only goal is to shed excess fat, as muscle is a calorie-burning furnace and will help you to quickly and permanently eliminate all excess body weight, even when sitting doing nothing. Any diet that restricts carbs in favour of high-protein or excessive fat intake won't permanently eliminate body fat. In fact, most of these dieters find themselves fatter after two to three months on carbohydrate-depriving diet plans.

EATING MORE CARBS IS NOT THE ANSWER

If you think that eating more carbohydrates is the answer, then I have to be honest with you, it's not! These diets produce an equally amazing effect as low-carb diets! In cases of high-carbohydrate ingestion, the body actually suppresses fat-burning hormones, preventing the release of stored calories. In fact, the only enzymes produced through a high-carbohydrate focus (insulin) are fat storing in nature. This means that, unless the calories are very low, you will gain fat!

Even if you were to sharply reduce calories, the excess carbohydrate concentration will continue to prevent the release of stored fat, but will gladly burn up muscle tissue (as protein content in such diet routines is extremely low). Thus, common diet philosophies concentrating on a high-carbohydrate, low-protein/fat basis provide results similar to that of low-carbohydrate/high-protein structures. Muscle is lost, and fat percentage increases!

GAINING WEIGHT HELPS BURN FAT

Muscle weight, that is. Gaining lean muscle mass speeds up your metabolism and, oh, by the way, it looks good and is also an excellent way to lose fat. Muscle requires more energy to maintain itself. Each pound of muscle you add to your body burns an extra 30 to 50 calories a day, so by adding ten pounds of muscle you burn an extra 500 calories per day. Try saying that about fat! That's why the Solitary Fitness programme incorporates both cardiovascular exercise and resistance training. Now do you see the meaning behind it all?

TRANS FATS – BAD FATS

Your body needs and can burn every kind of fat except one: trans fats, those mutant pseudo-nutrients created through the refining of healthy oils. They're found in most fried foods and processed baked goods. The red flag on the list of ingredients is 'partially hydrogenated vegetable oil'. Stay away from this junk if you're serious about weight loss and the health of your heart! You're much better off having one piece of chocolate, which contains healthy antioxidants, than making an entire meal out of foods with no redeeming value whatsoever.

REDUCING INSULIN SECRETION IS THE ANSWER

Bullet-proof abs, how many adverts use such phrases to get you hooked? Too many! No matter how bullet-proof your abs may be, they'll be hidden from view if they're beneath layers of ugly fat. In order to stop storing fat you must control insulin, but not by using today's popular 'no-carbohydrate' diet. One of the many keys to permanent weight loss is controlling the hormone 'insulin'. Proper calorific division, food selection and protein/carb percentages (where carbs are a part of the diet but properly balanced with protein), coupled with a potent exercise routine if you wish to accelerate results helps you reduce overall insulin secretion. It also causes an immediate release of stored calories (fat) into the bloodstream.

Insulin is essentially a fat-storage hormone and, if not properly manipulated through dietary variables, it will actually prevent fat loss, even on a low-calorie intake. This is the main reason why high-carbohydrate diet plans will never promote fat reduction, regardless of what many so-called 'dietary experts' have claimed. In addition, suppressing insulin reduces blood pressure and cholesterol readings, while preventing/curing diabetic symptoms, all of which are potentially deadly health issues.

STOMACH, HIPS, THIGHS, BUTTOCKS, LOVE HANDLES, ETC.

Contrary to popular belief, exercising a specific body part does not result in additional fat loss. You cannot spot reduce! The body has a predefined order of gaining and losing fat. This is genetic, which is why we all have different problem areas. We cannot modify this through exercise, diet or any other method. What we can do is force the body to burn stored fat through following a proper diet and as the body progresses through its own predefined order (arms, chest, thighs, waist, etc.), fat in those problem areas disappears!

If, for example, the stomach was the first area to gain considerable fat, you will find that it is also the last to lose fat, meaning you need to continue eliminating overall fat percentage through proper diet until the body begins to target the stomach region. You cannot change the body's natural, predetermined order of fat loss through exercise or any other method, so do not invest in any machine or technique that promises to target specific problem areas such as bullet-proof abs, solid thighs, lean hips or sleek arms. The key to solving any fat-loss dilemma is overall weight loss through a proper dietary focus.

STRESS MAKES YOU FAT

As surely as fast food will make you fat, so will stress. When you're chronically stressed, your adrenal glands continuously release cortisol, which in the long term causes your body to hold fat and redistribute it along the waistline. Stress is not a matter of being unhappy or irritable but is actually caused by a lot of the basic everyday chores that you in the free world have to do. If you're getting too little sleep and depending on caffeine and sugar for energy, your adrenal glands are probably working overtime and fattening you up. Your body also pumps cortisol during your long-distance travelling, when you're standing in a queue and when you're spending time with people you don't want to be with. Stress and its companion, cortisol, can be controlled with such simple efforts as thrice-weekly brisk walks of two or three miles. Or, even better, some Solitary Fitness workouts. Deep-breathing exercises, meditation and stretching regimes all provide relief.

WHAT ABOUT DIET PLANS?

Carbohydrate/low-protein, low-carbohydrate/high-protein, high-fat and calorie-restrictive diets are all ineffective in promoting permanent fat loss! What method will provide dramatic results? It takes no special drug, cream or machine to lose unwanted fat, but rather the knowledge to eat and exercise properly. This is the key to quick, permanent, healthy weight loss. Avoid weight-loss supplements and fancy electrical gadgets like the plague!

Once you know how to eat, you'll achieve your weight-loss goal without equipment, supplements or any external aids. If you wish to exercise for enhanced progress, then that's up to you.

BREAKFAST FUELS THE FAT-BURNING FURNACE

Wake up and smell the coffee! Three out of four people who lose a large amount of weight and keep it off eat breakfast every morning. It starts your metabolic furnace early on and it also reduces the risk of overeating and other poor food choices throughout the day. To keep the fat-furnace cooking, you should add extra, smaller meals to your day and not skip your regular ones. In addition to charging up your metabolism, this helps stabilise your blood sugar and minimises strain on your digestive system. Changing your eating patterns towards more frequent and smaller meals will also be of great assistance in keeping the furnace burning the fat!

SQUEEZE THE BEST OUT OF YOUR FOOD

One of the keys to shedding flab is getting more nutrition per calorie consumed so that you fill up quickly, stay satisfied longer and get all the nutrients you need despite eating fewer calories. When you eat a balance of nutritionally dense foods, including protein, healthy fats, unprocessed carbohydrates, fresh fruits and non-starchy vegetables, your food digests more slowly. This keeps your blood-glucose levels steady. Hunger signals result mainly from a drop in blood-glucose levels. Getting a good mix in your menu is easier at night when you have time to think about what you're cooking or ordering, but it's tougher when you're in a hurry.

AVOID FRANKENSTEIN-TYPE MACHINES

I've seen a machine comprised of electrodes that attach to muscles in the upper and lower body (electronic muscle stimulators). Makers of such units claim that electronic impulses miraculously 'massage' newfound muscle tone, simulating the impact of exercise while you sit comfortably in an easy chair watching your favourite television programme! These machines are absolutely useless in burning fat or enhancing tone, but the advertisements still make strong, convincing claims to the contrary.

Recently, I noticed that these same electrode-based products, proven false many years ago, have resurfaced, but with an interesting twist: they now wrap around your mid-section and are supposedly a cure for the bulging stomach! These false advertisements claim that a vibrating belt can transform your flabby belly into a sleek, slim mid-section. To put it mildly, these vibrating ab belts and muscle stimulators are a waste of your money, no different from supplements or the seemingly endless supply of abdominal toning devices available through mail-order companies! I can sit in my chair and sleep my way to a stunning mid-section! Unfortunately, you will wear the belt for several weeks, find absolutely no improvement in the appearance of your stomach and forget to return the product. Does this sound like you? The same concept applies to the electronic muscle stimulators. It's very sad, but endless lies and deceptions comprise this multi-billion-pound industry, and you've all fallen prey to their unethical advertising tactics!

MONITOR YOURSELF

Successful fat losers keep a tally. Consciously tracking your health-related behaviours by keeping exercise and food logs is a very effective way to keep yourself moving in the right direction. Make a note of these in written form – I do! Be sure to note periods of high and low energy and, when you come to study the logs, you'll realise why you experience these reactions and can adjust your eating and training sessions accordingly.

It's helpful to assess your progress using a scale, a measuring tape and/or a body-fat monitor. But give yourself every second or third day off. That will help keep you from becoming obsessive over constant minor weight fluctuations, most of which will be water in, or water out.

WALK OR JOG – EITHER

Q: Which burns more fat: walking or jogging?
A: Walking a mile burns about the same number of calories as a mile of jogging.

The important thing is to try to exercise at a level of

moderate intensity. This is equal to exercising at 60–85 per cent of your maximum heart rate. To determine your maximum heart rate, subtract your age from 220. Multiply that number by 0.6 or .85 in order to obtain the rate at 60–85 per cent.

NOT AN OVERNIGHT SUCCESS

Don't try to transform your entire lifestyle overnight. It's a recipe for failure. Those who have lived this way for a number of years, thereby damaging their metabolisms, will change all their habits and feel terrible because the new habits unmask the damage. Instead, change your diet first, and do it step by step. Find a way to manage stress (walking, yoga, meditation) and then wean yourself off any chemical dependencies, including sugar. Finally, build yourself a solid workout routine. If you start backsliding because your new lifestyle doesn't feel like you, then just remember, Rome wasn't built in a day!

EXCESS CARBS PRODUCE EXCESS INSULIN

Excess carbohydrates also cause vascular disease. The high-carbohydrate diet that is now so popular causes the pancreas to produce large amounts of insulin and, if this happens for many years in a genetically predisposed person, the insulin receptors throughout the body become resistant to insulin. Insulin's action is to drive glucose into the cells. This results in chronic hyperglycaemia, also called 'high blood sugar'. A large portion of this sugar is stored as fat, resulting in obesity. Excess insulin also causes hypertension and helps initiate the sequence of events in the arterial wall, which leads to arteriosclerosis and heart disease.

It's known that adult-onset diabetes is greatly benefited

by the adoption of a low-carbohydrate diet that's moderate in fat and which stresses the importance of a regular intake of sufficient protein. Excess fats damage the immune system through irradiation by free radicals during peroxidation of fats. Excess carbohydrates, known as eicosanoids, upset the hormonal system mentioned above and result in an imbalance favouring the type of eicosanoid (known as prostaglandins E-2 or PGE-2), which also suppresses the immune system. Thus, obesity is associated with a higher incidence of infection. So start changing your lifestyle now or you'll never make 100!

FOUR TYPES OF FAT

In human nutrition there are four different kinds of fat, which is categorised according to its saturation (the number of hydrogen atoms attached to the fat molecule). When a fat molecule contains the maximum number of hydrogen atoms ('saturated'), it is called hard fat because it remains hard at room temperature. If one pair of hydrogen atoms is missing, the molecule is said to be 'monounsaturated'. An example is olive oil. Monounsaturated fat is the healthiest, most easily digestible form of fat. If more than one pair of hydrogen atoms is missing, it is said to be 'polyunsaturated'. These are the thin oils commonly used for frying and for salad dressing.

Adding hydrogen atoms, which did not exist in nature, alters unsaturated vegetable fat: the fat molecule is 'hydrogenated'. Hydrogenation transforms the shape of a fatty acid to a 'trans' form. The molecule does not occur in nature and the body has difficulty digesting it. This is the problem with margarine – it contains hydrogenated, trans-fatty acids. Studies show this type of molecule to be more associated with artery disease than the saturated ('hard') fat found in butter. Hydrogenated fat is also commonly associated with junk food – crisps, biscuits, etc. It is very hard to digest and strongly linked to vascular disease.

There are one, maybe two fatty acids that cannot be manufactured by the body and must be consumed from outside sources. Linoleic acid is definitely necessary for human nutrition and it may be that linolenic acid also is necessary. Animal foods, except for fish and poultry, are low in linoleic acid, but they do meet human needs. Linoleic acid is abundant in vegetables and animal foods, and it is practically impossible to be in short supply of this nutrient unless starvation is also at your doorstep. With the exceptions of linoleic and linolenic acids, the body knows how to manufacture the fatty substances it needs. The body can cope with a relatively small intake of excess fats, though. What constitutes excess is in debate, but you can be sure that more than 40 per cent of your calories from fat constitute excess. To get an excess of fat in your diet, you must eat a junk food and/or animal source diet not properly balanced with plant-source food. If you do eat an excess of fat, the result is oxidation of these excess fats with the production of free radicals: molecules with an extra electron. Oxygen comes with four electrons in the common gaseous O_2 state, which is dissolved in body tissues and readily available for oxidation. When only three of these electrons are used, as is the case in fat breakdown, that leaves an extra electron. The result is the formation of the highly active and reactive hydroxyl radical (OH-). Your body is subjected to the damage caused by this extra electron.

The hydroxyl free radical must be distinguished from the oxide free radical. The action of the oxide free radical, unlike the hydroxyl free radical, is to activate enzymatic processes at the level of cellular mitochondria, the chemical labs of cellular metabolism. Hydroxyl free radicals are bad news for the body and must be neutralised. Oxides are invigorating and should be left to do their good work. Hydroxyl free radicals are neutralised well in the young body, which has an abundance of antioxidants, molecules that absorb and neutralise this extra electron. As we age, we have fewer and fewer antioxidants, and this makes an excess of fat in the diet even harder to handle, subjecting the body to the carcinogenic and degenerative effects of these highly reactive electrons. Taking oral antioxidants such as vitamins A, C and E can ameliorate this effect.

The association between excess fat and degenerative diseases, such as vascular heart disease and arthritis, is definitively established, as is the association between excess dietary fat and the development of a variety of cancers. Vascular disease, caused by the peroxidation of excess fats, also causes generalised vascular disease throughout the body, eventually causing kidney, pancreas and liver failure, as well as cerebrovascular clogging with resulting strokes. One of the worst things you can do is to switch from butter to margarine, which contains hydrogenated vegetable oil and is far more harmful to your body than fat from butter. Only the switch from excess to moderate levels of fat will get the job done.

SALT

Salt aids water retention, as does pork ... so be warned!

WEIGHT CHART FOR WOMEN

Weight in kilos (pounds) based on ages 25–59 with the lowest mortality rate (indoor clothing weighing 1.5kg/3lb and shoes with 2.5cm/1in heels).

HEIGHT	SMALL FRAME	MEDIUM FRAME	LARGE FRAME
1.47m 4ft 10in	46.2–50.3kg 118–131lb	49.4–54.8kg 102–111lb	53.5–59.4kg 109–121lb
1.50m 4ft 11in	46.7–51.2kg 120–134lb	50.3–55.7kg 103–113lb	54.4–60.7kg 111–123lb
1.52m 5ft	47.1–52.1kg 104–115lb	51.2–57.1kg 113–126lb	55.3–62.1kg 122–137lb
1.55m 5ft 1in	48–53.5kg 106–118lb	52.1–58.5kg 115–129lb	56.7–63.5kg 125–140lb
1.57m 5ft 2in	48.9–54.8kg 108–121lb	53.5–59.8kg 118–132lb	58–64.8kg 128–143lb
1.60m 5ft 3in	50.3–56.2kg 111–124lb	54.8–61.2kg 121–135lb	59.4–66.6kg 131–147lb
1.62m 5ft 4in	51.7–57.6kg 114–127lb	56.2–62.5kg 124–138lb	60.7–68.4kg 134–151lb
1.65m 5ft 5in	53–58.9kg 117–130lb	57.6–63.9kg 127–141lb	62.1–70.3kg 137–155lb
1.67m 5ft 6in	54.4–60.3kg 120–133lb	58.9–65.3kg 130–144lb	63.5–72.1kg 140–159lb
1.70m 5ft 7in	55.7–61.6kg 123–136lb	60.3–66.6kg 133–147lb	64.8–73.9kg 143–163lb
1.73m 5ft 8in	57.1–63kg 126–139lb	61.6–68kg 136–150lb	66.2–75.7kg 146–167lb
1.75m 5ft 9in	58.5–64.4kg 129–142lb	63–69.4kg 139–153lb	67.5–77.1kg 149–170lb
1.78m 5ft 10in	59.8–65.7kg 132–145lb	64.4–70.7kg 142–156lb	68.9–78.4kg 152–173lb
1.80m 5ft 11in	61.2–67.1kg 135–148lb	65.7–72.1kg 145–159lb	70.3–79.8kg 155–176lb
1.82m 6ft	62.5–68.4kg 138–151lb	67.1–73.4kg 148–162lb	71.6–81.1kg 158–179lb

WEIGHT CHART FOR MEN

Weight in kilos (pounds) based on ages 25–59 with the lowest mortality rate (indoor clothing weighing 2.2kg/5lb and shoes with 2.5cm/1in heels).

HEIGHT	SMALL FRAME	MEDIUM FRAME	LARGE FRAME
1.57m 5ft 2in	58–60.7kg 128–134lb	59.4–63.9kg 131–141lb	62.5–68kg 138–150lb
1.60m 5ft 3in	58.9–61.6kg 130–136lb	60.3–64.8kg 133–143lb	63.5–69.4kg 140–153lb
1.62m 5ft 4in	59.8–62.5kg 132–138lb	61.2–65.7kg 135–145lb	64.4–70.7kg 142–156lb
1.65m 5ft 5in	60.7–63.5kg 134–140lb	62.1–67.1kg 137–148lb	65.3–72.5kg 144–160lb
1.67m 5ft 6in	61.6–64.4kg 136–142lb	63–68.4kg 139–151lb	66.2–74.3kg 146–164lb
1.70m 5ft 7in	62.5–65.7kg 138–145lb	64.4–69.8kg 142–154lb	67.5–76.2kg 149–168lb
1.73m 5ft 8in	63.5–67.1kg 140–148lb	65.7–71.2kg 145–157lb	68.9–78kg 152–172lb
1.75m 5ft 9in	64.4–68.4kg 142–151lb	67.1–72.5kg 148–160lb	70.3–79.8kg 155–176lb
1.78m 5ft 10in	65.3–69.8kg 144–154lb	68.4–73.9kg 151–163lb	71.6–81.6kg 158–180lb
1.80m 5ft 11in	66.2–71.2kg 146–157lb	69.8–75.2kg 154–166lb	73.4–83.4kg 162–184lb
1.82m 6ft	67.5–72.5kg 149–160lb	71.2–77.1kg 157–170lb	74.3–85.2kg 164–188lb
1.85m 6ft 1in	68.9–74.3kg 152–164lb	72.5–78.9kg 160–174lb	76.2–87kg 168–192lb
1.88m 6ft 2in	70.3–76.2kg 155–168lb	74.3–80.7kg 164–178lb	78–89.3kg 172–197lb
1.90m 6ft 3in	71.6–78kg 158–172lb	75.7–82.5kg 167–182lb	79.8–91.6kg 176–202lb
1.93m 6ft 4in	73.4–79.8kg 162–176lb	77.5–84.8kg 171–187lb	82.1–93.8kg 181–207lb

CALCULATING YOUR FRAME SIZE

The following is the method used to calculate frame size:

1. Extend your arm out in front of your body, bending your elbow at a 90-degree angle to your body so that your forearm is parallel to it.

2. Keep your fingers straight and turn the inside of your wrist towards your body.

3. Place your thumb and index finger on the two prominent bones on either side of your elbow, then measure the distance between the bones with a tape measure or callipers.

4. Compare to the chart below, which lists elbow measurements for a medium frame. If your elbow measurement for your height is less than the amount listed, you are a small frame, and, if it is more than listed, you are a large frame.

ELBOW MEASUREMENTS FOR MEDIUM FRAME			
MEN	**ELBOW MEASUREMENT**	**WOMEN**	**ELBOW MEASUREMENT**
1.57–1.60m 5ft 2in–5ft 3in	6–7.2cm 2½–2⅞in	1.47–1.50m 4ft 10in–4ft 11in	5.7–6cm 2¼–2½in
1.62–1.70m 5ft 4in–5ft 7in	6.6–7.2cm 2⅝–2⅞in	1.52–1.60m 5ft–5ft 3in	5.7–6cm 2¼–2½in
1.73–1.80m 5ft 8in–5ft 11in	7–7.5cm 2¾–3in	1.62–1.70m 5ft 4in–5ft 7in	6–6.6cm /2⅜–2⅝in
1.82–1.90m 6ft–6ft 3in	7–5.3cm 2¾–2⅛in	1.73–1.80m 5ft 8in–5ft 11in	6–6.6cm 2⅜–2⅝in
1.93m 6ft 4in	7.2–8.2cm 2⅞–3¼in	1.82m 6ft	6–7cm 2½–2¾in

SOLITARY OILS

I dedicate this chapter to my late brother John Peterson RIP, pictured in Australian Army Band uniform. He died at his home in Australia at 9.10am on 3 March 2001 after a long and brave battle against cancer of the brain. Had I known about it at that time, then you bet I would have insisted he underwent flax-seed oil therapy! After a major operation to remove a malignant tumour he survived for some months. God rest you, John.

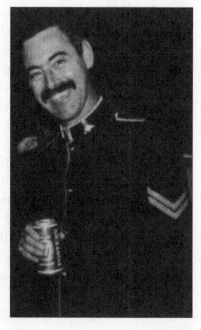

Just to show you how gullible people are, I'm gonna tell you a story about oil. Many years ago, an advert claimed to have a cure for male pattern baldness! Of course, if such an advertising claim was made today it would be met with scepticism, but back then it was a free for all and no such thing as the Advertising Standards Authority existed in the UK. The advert promised hair growth if you applied a Red Indian treatment ... coconut oil. I believe it sold by the tanker load! Now to the intelligent person this advertisement would start alarm bells ringing coz they don't have coconut trees on North American Indian Reservations! But, even though this contradictory advertisement was run, it still roped people in.

Dr Budwig began treating her patients by giving them a combination of high-quality flaxseed oil – which is rich in omega-3 oil – and quark, which is similar to cottage cheese or yoghurt in that it is rich in high-quality protein. If you can't find quark, yoghurt, cottage cheese, skimmed milk, soymilk or rice milk are good substitutes. By combining the protein with the oil, the oil becomes water soluble in the body and can be absorbed more readily. It can enter the smallest capillaries, dissolving undesirable fats and cleaning out the veins and arteries. This mixture also strengthens the heart, dissolves tumours and cures arthritis. It sounds like a lot to claim, but it really works. Dr Budwig worked with many patients who were terminally ill and some who had only hours to live. She gave them the combination of oil-protein plus organic foods, exercise, fresh air and used the healing powers of the sun to cure these hopeless cases.

The following is a quote from her book *Flax Oil As A*

True Aid Against Arthritis, Heart Infarction, Cancer And Other Diseases:

So here I am recommending certain oils to you, but without the hype and without any promises. All I will say is that I've studied the benefits of flaxseed oil (not flax oil) and my own findings make me satisfied that there are merits in what I'm about to reveal to you. But again I give you this caveat: I am not a doctor and I do not make any medical claims of a cure or remedy for medical problems. Always consult your own doctor on matters relating to medical problems before embarking on any type of homeopathic or other non-medical treatment.

The little plant on the left is one of the most miraculous plants on earth! It has been claimed to be a so-called cure for cancer and the subject of civil court actions against Dr Johanna Budwig, a biochemist and blood specialist from Germany, who has been treating cancer of all kinds with nothing but cottage cheese and flaxseed oil for over 16

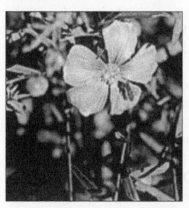 years. Dr Budwig says that people with cancer have blood that is low in omega-3 and omega-6 fatty acids and the blood has a greenish cast. Flaxseed oil is 56 per cent omega-3 and 16 per cent omega-6. It is believed that most people have blood that is 80 per cent deficient in omega-3

I often take very sick cancer patients away from hospital where they are said to have only a few days

left to live, or perhaps only a few hours. This is mostly accompanied by very good results. The very first thing that these patients and their families tell me is that, in the hospital, it was said that they could no longer urinate or produce bowel movements. They suffered from dry coughing without being able to bring up any mucous. Everything was blocked. It greatly encourages them when suddenly, in all these symptoms, the surface-active fats, with their wealth of electrons, start reactivating the vital functions and the patient immediately begins to feel better. It is very interesting to ask how this sudden change is possible. It has to do with the reaction patterns, with the character of electrons. I will return to these electrons later. In the last two years, I have come to be very fond of them. A friend of my work in Paris wrote to me: 'How wonderful it is that you have discovered the original birthplace of the electrons in seed oils to be the sun. That's how these connections are made!'

The conventional medical establishments are perplexed at her findings ... not surprising since billions of pounds and dollars could be lost in the sale of pharmaceutical anti-cancer drugs due to just one little plant! Oh, I forgot to mention that Dr Budwig was nominated seven times for the Nobel Prize and she goes on to say, 'This essential nutrient combination actually prevents and cures cancer.'

FLAXSEED OIL AND COTTAGE CHEESE

Doctors had attempted to treat patients with sources of omega-3 but had not been consistently successful. Dr Budwig's research found that, in order for these fatty acids to be fully available to the body, they must be tied to a particular protein, the best source of which is cottage cheese. Depending on the severity of the condition, she had her patients use three to six tablespoons of flaxseed oil a day, with at least 125g (4oz) or half a cup of cottage cheese per day. Dr Budwig recommends that the oil and the cottage cheese be thoroughly mixed before they are eaten.

I have realised that an excellent approach would be to mix however many tablespoons of flaxseed oil one plans to use each day in a bowl with at least half a cup of cottage cheese and some fruit, such as crushed pineapple or frozen strawberries. Put it in the refrigerator and eat a portion of it at different times during the day. Flaxseed oil is increasingly available in health-food stores, though it must be kept fresh, cold and out of direct light. It will keep for up to a year in the freezer and four months in a refrigerator but only three weeks at room temperature, so be careful!

In 1994 Dr Budwig said, 'I have the answer to cancer but American doctors won't listen. They come here and observe my methods and are impressed. Then they want to make a special deal so they can take it home and make a lot of money. I won't do it, so I'm blackballed in every country.'

Her methods have incurred the wrath of the establishment and she is passed over, especially upsetting is her refusal to use radiation or chemotherapy.

Here, I will add a word of warning: I don't know much about diabetes, but I have learned that one type is caused by a lack of omega-3 fatty acid. Where that is the case, the use of flaxseed oil for cancer has also taken care of the diabetes. I have read that a number of times.

DOSAGE

The recommended dosage for health maintenance is one tablespoon of flaxseed oil to ¼ cup cottage cheese per

45.3kg (100lb) body weight. In her book, Dr Budwig says she uses three tablespoons of oil a day and sometimes up to six for people who are very seriously ill. These dosages are just suggestions and in no way constitute medical advice. Be sure that the oil you purchase is cold pressed, i.e. never heated in the processing. Make sure it is refrigerated or frozen as much as possible. Heat of any kind destroys the value of the oil. I do not recommend the capsules as it takes approximately 14 of them to equal one tablespoon of oil and also because they are often stored on warm shelves for periods of time. DO NOT USE THE OIL FOR COOKING! Heating the oil destroys its healing qualities!

All over the world discoveries of miraculous cures for cancer have taken place and the claim to these remissions

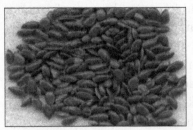 and recoveries has been attributed to flaxseed oil. Fewer people have had greater impact on the medical community and modern nutritional science than Dr Budwig.

TIP

If you have something caught in your eye, place a flax seed on a moist cotton bud tip. Positioning it under the upper eyelid will help reduce the pain and lubricate the object, allowing it to move into the corner of the eye where it can be removed.

THE BENEFITS OF FLAX SEEDS

- Flax seeds contain a high-quality protein.
- They are rich in soluble fibre. The combination of the oil and the fibre makes flaxseeds an ideal laxative.
- Vitamins B-1, B-2, C, E and carotene are in flax seeds.

The seeds also contain iron, zinc and trace amounts of potassium, magnesium, phosphorus, calcium and vitamin E and carotene, which aid the metabolism of the oil.

- Flax seeds contain over 100 times more of a phytonutrient known as lignin than wheat bran, buckwheat, rye, millet, oats and soybeans. Lignins have received a lot of attention because of possible anti-cancer properties, especially in relation to breast and colon cancer. They seem to flush excess oestrogen out of the body, thereby reducing the incidence of oestrogen-linked cancers, such as breast cancer. Besides anti-tumour properties, lignins also seem to have antibacterial, antifungal and antiviral properties.

Because they contain some protein, fibre, vitamins and minerals and lignins, flax seeds are more nutritious than their oil. Yet, for practical purposes, most consumers find it simpler to use the oil for its omega-3 fatty acids without having to bother grinding the seeds. But, nutritionally speaking, it's worth the trouble to grind fresh flax seeds (say, in a coffee grinder), and sprinkle them as a seasoning on salads or cereals or mix them into muffins. When buying seeds, be sure they are whole and not split (splitting exposes the inner seed to light and heat and decreases the nutritional value). Or buy pre-ground flax seeds that are available as flaxseed meal. About four tablespoons of flaxseed meal will yield about 6gm of protein and 8gm of fibre.

HEALTH-PROMOTING PROPERTIES OF FLAX

Flaxseed oil, flax seeds and the omega-3 fatty acids they contain are good for your health. Here are some of the ways flax helps your body:

- Flax promotes cardiovascular health. The ultra-high levels of omega-3 fatty acids lower LDL (bad) cholesterol levels. Fish oils and algae are also good sources of essential fatty acids.
- It promotes the health of the colon. Flax has anti-cancer properties and, as a natural lubricant and a rich source of fibre, it lowers the risk of constipation.
- Supplements of flax can boost immunity. One study showed that school children who had less than a teaspoon of flaxseed oil a day had fewer and less severe respiratory infections than children not taking flaxseed oil supplements.
- Flax provides fats that are precursors for brain building. This is especially important at the stage of life when a child's brain grows the fastest, which is in the uterus and during infancy. A prudent mum should consider supplementing her diet with a daily tablespoon of flaxseed oil during her pregnancy and while breastfeeding.
- Flax promotes healthy skin. It has been used as a dietary supplement for patients who seem to have dry skin or eczema, or whose skin is particularly sun-sensitive.
- The severity of diabetes may be lessened because flax stabilises blood-sugar levels.
- Flax fat can be slimming. Fats high in essential fatty acids, such as flax, increase your metabolic rate, helping to burn the excess, unhealthy fats in the body. Eating the right kind of fat gives you a better fighting chance as your body stores the right amount of fats. This is called thermogenesis, a process in which specialised fat cells throughout the body (called brown fat) click into high gear and burn more fat when

activated by essential fatty acids, especially gamma-linolenic acid (GLA). You might have noticed that you crave less fat overall when you get enough healthy fats. A daily supplement of omega-3 fatty acids may be an important part of weight-control programmes.

USING FLAXSEED OIL

1. Don't use flaxseed oil for cooking. Oils high in essential fatty acids are not good for cooking. In fact, heat can turn these healthy fats into harmful ones. Add flaxseed oil to foods after cooking and just before serving.
2. Flax has many virtues, but it also has one vice: it turns rancid quickly. Healthy fats spoil quickly (olive oil is an exception to the rule). The fats with a long shelf-life are the hydrogenated shortenings, which of course are bad for you. To prevent spoilage, follow these tips:
* Purchase only refrigerated flaxseed oil stored in black containers.
* Keep your oil in the refrigerator with the lid on tight. Minimise exposure to heat, light and air.
* Because the oil is likely to turn rancid within six weeks of pressing, buy flaxseed oil in smaller containers 250–375g (8–12oz) depending on how fast you use it.
3. Taken with a meal, flaxseed oil can actually increase the nutritional value of other foods. Research shows that adding flaxseed oil to foods rich in sulphated amino acids, such as cultured dairy products (i.e. yoghurt), vegetables of the cabbage family and animal, seafood and soy proteins help the essential fatty acids become incorporated into cell membranes. Mixing flaxseed oil with yoghurt helps emulsify the oil, improving its digestion and metabolism by the body.
4. Flaxseed oil works best in the body when it's taken

237

along with antioxidants, such as vitamins E, carotene and other nutrients, such as vitamin B6 and magnesium. But the main thing is that you get it down your neck!

QUARK

Definition: (qwark) a soft, unripened cheese with the texture and flavour of sour cream. Quark comes in two versions: low fat and non-fat. Though the calories are the same (35 per 25g/1oz), the texture of low-fat quark is richer than that of low-fat sour cream. It has a milder flavour and richer texture than low-fat yoghurt, too. Quark can be used to top baked potatoes as a sour cream and in a variety of dishes including cheesecakes, dips, salads and sauces. You can substitute cottage cheese or yoghurt for quark.

Did you know that a third of high cholesterol is caused by an omega-3 fatty acid deficiency? A daily tablespoon of omega-3-rich flaxseed oil is a must!

FLAXSEED BENEFITS PROSTATE CANCER ... SO THEY SAY

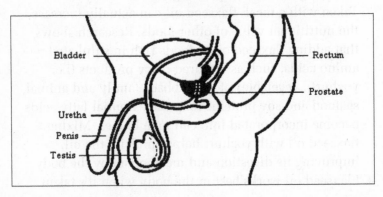

In a study, it was found that after five weeks prostate cancer patients who added about three tablespoons of ground flaxseed to their daily diet had more slowly dividing cells (tumour) and a greater rate of tumour cell

BREAST CANCER

Breast cancer happens when some of the cells in the breast start to grow out of control. When this happens, a cancerous growth begins to appear somewhere inside the breast. Sometimes it is in the lobules, but often it is in the lining of the ducts. If it isn't treated, cancer cells from the breast can spread to other parts of the body.

There are about 20 different kinds of breast cancer. Some are more dangerous than others: either they grow faster or they're more likely to spread. Below are the added risk factors:

1. More than half the women who are diagnosed with breast cancer are over 65.
2. Having a close relative, like a mother, sister or daughter (or more than one), who was diagnosed with breast cancer – especially when fairly young (under 45).
3. Not having children.
4. Having your first child when you're over 30.
5. Drinking excessive amounts of alcohol.
6. Women whose periods start when they're very young or whose periods stop later than usual.

WHAT ARE THE SYMPTOMS OF BREAST CANCER?

Women's breasts change throughout their lives, from the time they start to grow in their late childhood or early teens to when their periods stop in their forties or fifties. While women are having their periods, they change every month as well and they may get swollen and tender. The nipple may change in colour, shape or size. Breast changes to look out for – all the way to your armpits – include:

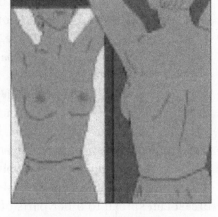

1. Pain in part of your breast.
2. Getting dimples in your breast.
3. A change in the shape, feel or colour of the skin of a breast.
4. Anything coming out of your nipple without squeezing, except breast milk.
5. A lump, or a feeling of lumpiness or thickness somewhere in your breast.
6. A nipple that turns in when it used to stick out (a nipple that's always been turned in is nothing to worry about).

These changes don't usually mean you have breast cancer. Nine times out of ten, it's a change that's normal for you and the way you're made. But, if you do experience any of these changes, see your doctor just to make sure.

BREAST SELF-EXAMINATION

Lying down: Lie down with a pillow under your right shoulder, bend your elbow and place your right hand behind your head. Use the finger pads (the top third of each finger) of the middle three fingers on your left hand to feel for any lumps or thickening.

In the shower: You can also do your breast examination in the shower. Raise your right arm and, with a soapy left hand, check your right breast. Your hands will glide over the wet skin, making it easy to check how your breast feels. Use the same technique as described above. Repeat with the left breast. Feel for lumps using a firm, rubbing motion, without lifting the fingers. You can do this in one of three ways:

• Use a wedge pattern
• Follow a circular pattern
• Use an up and down pattern.

Follow the same method every time. It will help you to make sure you've gone over the entire breast.

In front of a mirror: You can also check your breasts standing in front of a mirror. Look for changes in your breasts – dimpling or puckering of the skin, thickness or a lump, and any change in size or shape. Check the nipple for signs of fluid or bloodstained discharge, redness or swelling.

TESTICULAR CANCER

The most common symptom of cancer of the testis is a small (although it can be any size), hard lump in one of the testicles. Some men notice a swelling, a feeling of heaviness and accumulation of fluid or a dull pain in a testicle, or in the scrotum. These warning signs do not necessarily mean cancer is present. Other conditions can cause similar symptoms. Men who notice any of these symptoms should see their doctor immediately to rule out or confirm the possibility of cancer. After examining a questionable lump or swelling, the doctor may order appropriate tests and then recommend removing the lump for examination under a microscope. Cancer cells can look different than normal cells.

IS TESTICULAR CANCER DANGEROUS?

People worry a good deal about cancer today and rightly so. If allowed to run its course unchecked, cancer usually kills! The good news is that many forms of cancer can now be cured, provided they are detected early enough. Fortunately, testicular cancer has a very high rate of cure especially when detected early and when it is appropriately treated with surgery, chemotherapy and, for certain types, radiation therapy. Regular physical examinations, self-examinations of the testes and attentiveness to the warning signs of testicular cancer give you a good chance to catch it early enough to cure it. But, if all else fails, then get that flaxseed oil into your system!

TESTICULAR SELF-EXAMINATION

Men should routinely examine their testicles once a month for early warning signs of cancer. The earlier you catch the disease, the greater the likelihood of a cure without it spreading to other regions of the body. A monthly examination familiarises a man with the normal size, feel and look of his testicles. Ideally, self-examination takes place after a hot bath or shower. The heat relaxes the scrotum and skin, making examination easier and more effective.

Standing up: The man should begin by standing naked in front of a full-length mirror to check the appearance of the scrotum for noticeable swellings or lumps. Next, he should gently roll each testicle between his thumb and the index and middle fingers of both hands. Any hard lumps should be reported immediately to a physician. If the lumps are not cancerous, you will feel reassured and, if they are, early treatment increases the chances of a cure.

PROSTATE GLAND

Unpleasant as it may be or seem (and I've had it done!), the digital rectal examination (DRE) is a man's first line of defence against cancer of the prostate gland. The doctor checks for palpable abnormalities in the prostate through the thin wall of the rectum.

WHAT CAN I DO TO PREVENT CANCER?

1. Don't smoke.
2. Consume flaxseed oil.
3. Leave sugar out of your diet.
4. Cut down on red meat, but not entirely.
5. Veggies and fruits also contain plant chemicals, which fight cancer, and these are called phytochemicals.
6. Limit your fat intake by drinking skimmed milk and eating lean cuts of meat; also taking the skin off chicken and turkey.
7. Fibre-rich foods like whole grains, beans, fruits and vegetables with their skin on and seeds protect you against colon cancer.
8. Some forms of cancer are linked to obesity, so maintain a healthy weight by getting a minimum of 30 minutes' physical activity every day.
9. Eat your veggies and fruits – at least five servings a day. They contain nutrients called antioxidants (like beta carotene and vitamin C), which protect body cells from cancer.
10. The following oils are excellent for your health:

- **Borage oil:** Borage has been used in connection with the following conditions: eczema, infantile dermatitis and rheumatoid arthritis. The oil is extracted from the seed of the blue star-shaped flowers and its active component, gamma linoleic acid (GLA), has drawn the interest of researchers. The majority of the early studies done on GLA, dating back to the late 1940s, were conducted with evening primrose oil. Borage seed oil is the richest source of gamma linolenic acid (GLA) and contains 20–26 per cent GLA.

- **Coconut oil (not for baldies):** Coconut oil was fed as 7 per cent of energy to patients recovering from heart attacks. The patients showed a greater improvement than those untreated and no difference compared to those treated with corn or safflower oils. Populations consuming coconut oil have low rates of heart disease, maybe because of its antiviral and anti-microbial characteristics.

- **Hemp oil (cannabis):** Hemp seed is the richest source of essential fatty acids (EFAs) in the plant kingdom and it contains a relatively low percentage of saturated fats. The EFAs in the oil and seeds promote cellular growth, healthy skin, hair and eyes; they also aid in immune response, disease prevention, weight control and even in cognitive functions. The human brain is 60 per cent fat and therefore the EFAs are vital to its proper function and good health. EFAs are also the raw material the body needs to produce hormones, the body's communication network for cellular activity. Hemp oil supports the body's detoxification process due to the fact that the LA (linoleic acid) and ALA (alpha- linolenic acid) have the ability to carry toxic substances to the surface of the skin, intestinal tract,

244

kidneys and lungs, where they can be eliminated from the body.

- **Fish oil:** Most of the salmon you eat is farmed. Only fish from the oceans contain a good source of omega-3 essential fatty acids. Farmed fish usually doesn't contain much omega-3.

HOW TO LOOK THE SAME AGE AS YOU DO NOW IN TEN YEARS' TIME

> **Thyme oil (white):** An essential oil, meaning it contains the essence of thyme leaves. Locked into this oil is one of the biggest secrets that will blow all the face-cream manufacturers into orbit! The name of this oil gives a clue to what it can magically do for you! In small amounts, thyme oil (Thymus vulgaris) can be used externally as a fragrance or with other massage oils, or as a seasoning. It works as bactericide, antiseptic, anti-microbial, astringent, antispasmodic, antitoxic, diuretic, anti-fungal, insecticide, tonic and an immune stimulant. Do not use if you are pregnant or have high blood pressure or a child. Seek professional advice for internal use!

I've left this particular piece right until the very end, so you can find it again when you want to show your friends or use it for reference purposes! An agricultural university in Scotland stumbled on this little-known secret when researching the thyme plant. Just as the plant is named 'thyme', the oil itself has the ingredients to lock you into time. Mixing 1 per cent of thyme oil with 99 per cent of carrier oil will give you the required mixture.

Warning: Undiluted thyme oil strips the skin from your face – do not attempt to apply it directly to bare flesh! Seek

the guidance of a professional when getting this mixed.
After a few months of applying the mixture every morning,
you will notice the difference ... I can't wait to get out there
to apply my own mix ... Go for it, girls and boys!

SOLITARY TIPS

- **Fast:** Every so often, say once a month, go two days
  without food and drink lots of fluids (I just do water,
  but you should have fruit juices too – I'd do juices as
  well if I were outside). Anyway, the reason for this is
  simple … you need to clean out and there is no better
  way to do it. If you can't survive without something to
  eat, just have fruit. Yeah, clear out the filth that lies in
  the gut and you'll feel lighter and faster and healthier.
  I also believe by doing this you will prevent stomach
  or bowel cancer ever happening. Follow with a good
  inner cleanse, as mentioned in Solitary Cleanse
  chapter. But seek medical advice first.
- **Jogging:** Try to run or jog on grass as it's less damaging
  to your joints and I say good sprints beat any long-term
  jogging. One day that sprint may save your life but a
  long jog might get you in trouble! Still, do what suits
  you best. You may be built for a marathon, so go for it!

Never do nothing you don't enjoy! That's my No. 1 belief. Enjoy your fitness – why do it otherwise?

- **Toes & Fingers:** People neglect these, but hell, you may need them one day to get you out of trouble and you must look after them! Tie string around your toes and also to a light weight (1–21/2kg/2–51/2lb is plenty). Or place a bag of sugar in a sock or bag. Just lift the weight up and down without moving your legs too much, just enough to feel the pain! To exercise your fingers, get a bucket of sand and keep stabbing your straight fingers into it; work up to using tiny pebbles. Obviously I can't do this – sure I miss it, but I do other things instead. I jab into crumpled blankets, sheets and towels.

- **Jaw:** Get a soft ball or something wrapped in cloth. Put it in your mouth and bite hard. Hold for 60 seconds, rest for 60 seconds and bite again for 60 seconds! Do this ten times – it strengthens the jaw.

- **Lungs:** People forget about lungs … You can't do much without them, so work on them! This is a good exercise. Get a ping-pong ball, put it on a table (save your back) and keep blowing it up against a wall. Don't let it stop, it will keep hitting the wall and coming back. Also, do lots of sucking in air (keep it down). Air is food for your lungs. Treat your body well and look after it coz you won't get another one. Love your body: respect it, coz if you don't then nobody else will!

- **Bite:** There's a lot of boredom in solitary! If you let it get to you, you'll go mad so invent exercises such as filling a pillowcase with books, boots, sheets, curtains, etc. so you have a decent weight. Bite into the case and squat lift down. Sounds easy, eh? Well, after 100 times you feel your jaw, neck, back and legs – it works miracles plus you have the best-ever bite! Remember your jaw has muscles that need working!

- **Mattress:** Place a mattress up on your shoulders and squat with it. Also use it as a punch bag or place it on your back and it's good for step-ups.
- **Reflexes:** A bar of soap is good for the reflexes. Chuck it up in the air to bounce off your bicep and then catch it. It's good for the reflexes, speed and accuracy. Now try it while you're in the bath or shower – it works the hand to eye co-ordination.
- **Balance:** Get two big books (Bibles or encyclopaedias are best). Balance them on your head and walk up and down. Squat and turn – it's all good for the equilibrium, all good for posture!
- **Grip:** Take an empty shampoo bottle and squeeze it. It's good for the grip.
- **Forearms:** This is good for dynamic stretching. Get a stick, tie a rope around the centre and put a large, heavy paint tin on the other end of the rope. Hold the stick in front of you and now start to wind the stick with both wrists (the can should be rising like a lift). Let it down and wind it back up again.
- **Handstand:** Drink a cup of water upside down while doing a handstand. Also learn to pick things up with your mouth, spit them out and pick up more – all upside down.

There are some things I do that I would never say, coz I don't want to be responsible for injuring people, plus some of my things are only for madmen! After all, we are special people.

MAKE A START!

Look, some of you are grossly out of shape, you're totally out of condition, life has smothered you! Bad diets, drink, fags, drugs and bad posture ... basically, you're full of shit! So get a grip ... coz it's rotting your life away! Try some of these tips:

- **Eyes:** Start by looking at the wall and then focus in on something – a clock for instance. Now, without moving your head, start to focus in at the frame of the clock, then focus in on the pointers, and then focus in on something on the pointers ... Hold for a few seconds and work your way back out. Do this ten times.

- **Extra energy:** Tired during a workout? Have a bite on a chocolate bar to give you an energy rush for a short while.

- **Fat burning:** Half an hour before your workout, have a small cup of black coffee.

- **Muscle pain:** A couple of teaspoons of bicarbonate of soda in a glass of water take the morning-after pain away.

- **Stomach cancer:** Green tea is richer than most fruits in antioxidant compounds known as flavonoids and polyphenols.

- **Muscle cramps:** Bananas are rich in potassium and will stave them off.

- **Prevent colds:** The beta carotene in mangoes, papaya, cantaloupe and eggs boost immunity, while the enzymes limonene and glucarase (found in citrus fruits) can speed toxins from your body.

- **Salt:** Cut it out of your diet and monitor foodstuffs for it!

- **Eating food:** Chew slowly and don't drink fluids with meals as it dilutes your digestive juices.

- **Eating out:** Order a child's portion.

- **Food:** Generally, the darker the food, the more nutrients in it.
- **Sugar:** Replace with barley malt, grape sugar, dextrose, fructose, glucose, honey or lactose.
- **Cooking:** Buy a pressure cooker or stir-fry to keep vitamins in food. Boiling kills vitamins.
- **Garlic:** Crush it, don't cut it!
- **Orange:** Peel it! Don't cut it or you kill up to 50 per cent of the vitamin C in it.
- **Protein:** When training, 1gm of protein per pound of bodyweight is needed. Spread it out over six meals per day.
- **Amino Acids:** To help convert protein into muscle you need an intake of amino acids. Soybeans have an abundant amount of all nine essential amino acids.
- **Alcohol:** Drink plenty of non-alcoholic fluids after a drinking session, otherwise you'll dehydrate.
- **Vitamins:** Top up daily on vitamin C and the entire list of B vitamins as they are all water-soluble, which means you cannot store them.
- **Daily diet:** A healthy diet means variety and eating foods from all five food groups – grains, vegetables, fruits, milk products and meats.
- **Goodies:** Now and again have a binge or you'll crack up!
- **Fibre:** If you're really hungry and desperate, eat some fruit.
- **Menstrual cycle:** Women, top up on iron during this time!

HANDSTAND PRESS-UPS

Begin by doing the handstand against the wall. Stay about two feet away from the wall whilst outing your hands flat on the floor. Throw your weight forward, re-membering to keep the arms locked! Kick your feet upwards and, eventually, get them against the wall. When you're in the position, arch your back to keep the balance aimed at the wall.

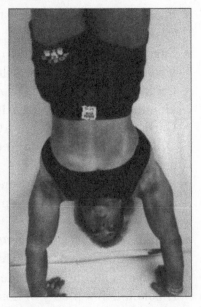

Don't be put off by the fumbling around and falling over. Eventually when you feel confident, take your whole weight on arms. You have to keep your arms straight in this particular exercise. I know I've said not to lock them out in other exercises, but this one is the exception.

Integrate this into your Solitary Fitness routine. Eventually do handstands press-ups. Remember to keep your back arched and be very careful with this exercise! Seek the advice of a doctor before you perform it!

SOLITARY
EXTRAS

The giant Brian Cockerill is a mountain of a man. He's probably the only man around who's turned down an invite to compete in Britain's Strongest Man competition. His exploits within the underworld of northern England are legendary ... no wonder I chose Brian to fill in for me and help demonstrate some of the little extras I've added.

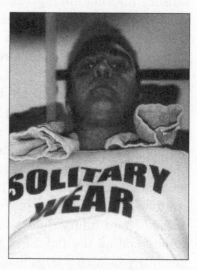

To begin with, I want to give you a short breakdown on why I advise you to stretch ... I don't want to bore you too much with technical details so I'll be as quick as I can.

THE GOLDEN GOLGI TENDON

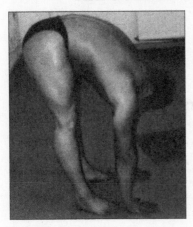
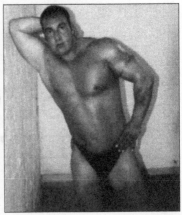

Muscles contain receptors called spindles and Golgi (named after a man) tendon organs. These provide sensory information regarding changes in the length and tension of the muscle. The main function of the spindles is to respond to the stretch in a muscle and, through reflex action, to initiate a stronger contraction to reduce this stretch.

Impulses from the Golgi tendon organs cause reflex relaxation of the muscle and its opposing muscle. When the actual stretch occurs, the spindles resist. If the stretch is held longer than six seconds, the Golgi tendon organs respond by allowing the muscle to reflexively relax. This lengthens the muscle and allows it to remain in a stretched position for a long period, reducing the possibility of injury due to the stretching. Here, Brian is demonstrating the flat hand to the floor technique. This flexibility in such a large man should give you some hope of doing the same. It's a great exercise to help enlarge the muscle during leg workouts.

The purpose of a stretching programme is to relax the

muscle and work it through the necessary range of motion. Stretching a muscle the wrong way, or at the wrong time can activate the stretch reflex causing the muscle to contract and become tighter rather than relaxed. This should be done after a muscle has been warmed up. Do not stretch immediately after a long run or strenuous workout when your muscles are apt to be fatigued and dehydrated. Here, Brian demonstrates how even a bare wall can be used to get the maximum from your stretches. Push and hold!

Set aside a separate period three to five times per week for a complete stretching routine of the exercises shown in this chapter and the Solitary Stretch chapter, which should take about 20 minutes.

FOUR TYPES OF STRETCH

Stretching is done to relax the muscles and the connective tissue. The connective tissue needs 20 seconds to relax and relaxing the muscles takes about two minutes.

- **Ballistic Stretching:** The old 'bounce, bounce, bounce' stretches that actually make the muscles shorter and tighter by activating the stretch reflex. They have been found to contribute to the risk of small muscle tears, soreness and injury – avoid them!

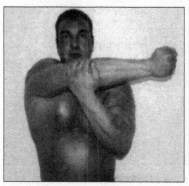

- **Static Stretching::** This is a slow, gradual stretch through the muscle's full range of motion until resistance is felt. It should be done slowly and carefully to the point of a slight pull or slight discomfort and should not be painful!

- **Proprioceptive Neuromuscular Facilitation (PNF) stretching:** This is more easily called the 'hold–relax' method of stretching which involves a contraction of the muscle followed by a relaxation and a stretch. The tightening 'fools' the stretch reflex, activating the Golgi tendon organ. This helps the muscle to relax before the actual stretch begins and allows you to stretch the muscle further.

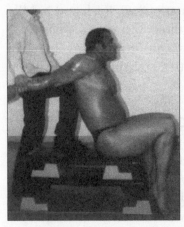

- **Enforced Prolonged Stretching:** The no-holds barred stretch! This is the only real way to induce muscle size. When the stretch is at its point of maximum resistance it has to be forcibly held either by the assistance of someone helping or by the use of an assister, such as a wall or some heavy object.

GET THE BEST FROM THE STRETCH

The stretches already shown can either be done statically without the contraction phase or using the PNF method

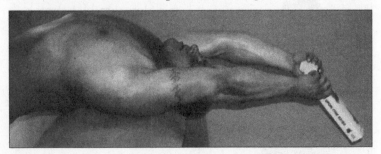

Do a pullover with a heavy object and allow it to stretch your chest, as above.

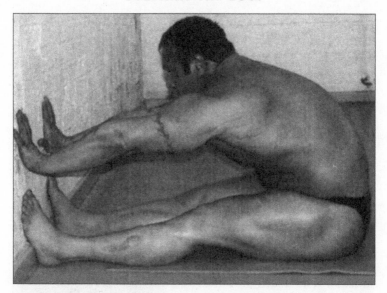

Push the wall away and hold.

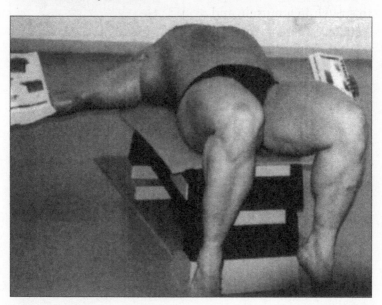

Books can be great... stretch!

with the contractions, followed by Enforced Prolonged Stretching. Contractions are achieved by tightening the muscle, not actually moving it.

FLEXIBILITY

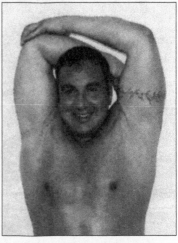

Lack of flexibility restricts the range of motion and may limit the extent of energy transfers. Muscles contain receptors called spindles and Golgi tendon organs that provide sensory information regarding changes in the length and tension of the muscle. The main function of the spindles is to respond to stretch in a muscle and to initiate a stronger contraction to reduce this stretch through reflex action. The stretch reflex mainly responds to voluntary movements and maintains upright posture.

As I have previously mentioned, your muscles are encased in a material that has a molecular structure which makes it stronger than steel! By stretching the muscles, you are stretching the protective material, thereby encouraging the muscle to expand naturally.

MAKE THE STRETCH BECOME AN EXERCISE

Get a book from the library that shows you the correct stretching methods you should employ. In such a small book as this, it is impossible to fit in everything you need to master. Stretching is the key to defining your body and allowing your muscles to grow.

ADVANCED ABS – LE CRUNCH

The Crunch is the most fundamental exercise for the abs. Do it on a flat surface to protect your lower back from injury. To start, lie flat on your back with your butt on the floor and with a slight bend in your knees with your feet about 0.6m (2ft) apart and flat on the floor. Cross your hands over your upper chest and tilt your pelvis to slowly curl your upper body towards your knees. Blow out as you curl your torso up and inhale as you lower your torso back down. Isolate your abs during this movement. The effort required to curl your torso up should come exclusively from your abs. Don't pull yourself up with your arms behind your neck and don't use your momentum to swing yourself up. When you've completely curled your upper body, slowly lower down.

MAKE IT HURT!

If it takes you 100 crunches before your abs begin to burn, then you're wasting your time. Your abs should be fatigued at no more than 20 to 25 reps. If they aren't, you need to add weights to your exercise and work on contracting the muscles tightly for each rep. Focus on how hard you can contract the abdominal muscles.

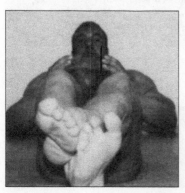

CRUNCH TWISTS

Add a twist to the movement to work your obliques. As you curl your upper body up towards your knees, twist one shoulder so it points to the opposite knee. Alternate the shoulder to the opposite knee to work both sides of your obliques.

LEGS RAISED CRUNCH

Perform the Legs Raised Crunch the same way you would a regular crunch, except this time raise your legs off the floor, keep your knees bent and cross your ankles. This movement will help isolate your abs even more.

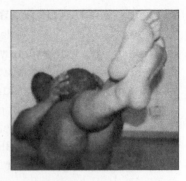

WEIGHTED CRUNCH

To perform a Weighted Crunch, hold a weight such as a medicine ball (pick one up from a second-hand shop) on your chest before you crunch.

A GREAT AB BLASTER!

Place your elbows directly under your shoulders to pick your shoulders and chest off the floor as shown. You're in

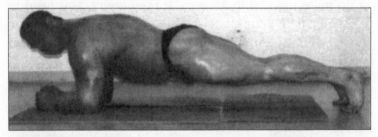

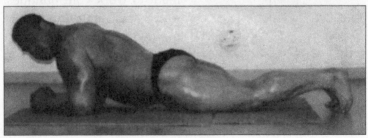

a board-like position, resting on toes and forearms. Tighten your abdominal muscles to prevent your back from sagging or arching. Hold for five to ten seconds and then lower as shown.

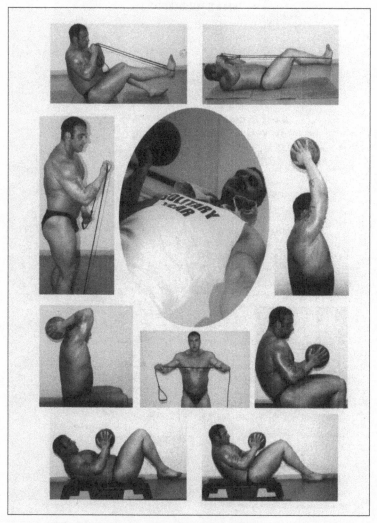

It's amazing what you can do with a ball and a rope!

THE KRAY'S

By Charlie Bronson

"MAX RESPECT"

Charlie, Ronnie and Reggie
Men of Honour, Men of Respect, Men of Rock
Legends in their own Lifetime
Icons in death, Myths in years to come
Never forgotten, who can ever forget the Kray's?
They were the cream of the crop, the dog's Bollocks
Who Said? History Say's, that's what Say's
Real life Facts, Reality
So who's taken their place?
Make me Laugh, Come on and tell me!
Punk Drug Gangs, Yardie Yobos,
When the Kray's passed on
There era went with them, It all ended
You'll never see the likes again, they had it all
Style, Charisma, Strength, Loyalty, Honour
They were Fearless, Powerful but Respected
They helped a lot of people
Old folks homes, Children's homes, Boxing clubs, Hospitals
There were no muggers on their Plot
Even burglars got sorted out
THE KRAY LAW
Judge, Jury, and Executioners
Right or Wrong
But the streets were Safe
Bethnal Green was alive with laughter
Ask the old folk there
Was it better then, or better now?
The Kray's died how they lived

MEN OF RESPECT